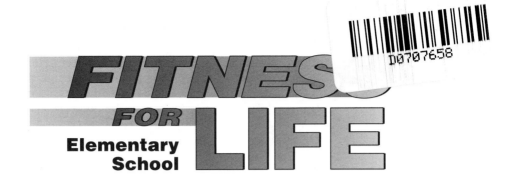

FITNESS FOR LIFE

Elementary School

Guide for Wellness Coordinators

Charles B. Corbin

Guy C. Le Masurier

Dolly D. Lambdin

Meg Greiner

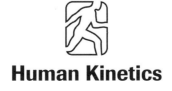

Human Kinetics

Library of Congress Cataloging-in-Publication Data

Fitness for life : elementary school guide for wellness coordinators / Charles B. Corbin ... [et al.].
    p. cm.
  Includes bibliographical references.
  ISBN-13: 978-0-7360-8718-6 (soft cover)
  ISBN-10: 0-7360-8718-4 (soft cover)
  1. Physical fitness for children--Study and teaching (Elementary) I. Corbin, Charles B.
  GV443.F528 2010
  372.86--dc22
                            2009043017

ISBN-10: 0-7360-8718-4 (print)
ISBN-13: 978-0-7360-8718-6 (print)

The Web addresses cited in this text were current as of January 2010, unless otherwise noted.

Acquisitions Editor: Scott Wikgren; **Developmental Editor:** Ray Vallese; **Assistant Editor:** Derek Campbell; **Copyeditor:** Mary Rivers; **Permission Manager:** Dalene Reeder; **Graphic Designer:** Fred Starbird; **Graphic Artist:** Denise Lowry; **Cover Designer:** Keith Blomberg; **Photographer (cover):** © Human Kinetics; **Photographer (interior):** © Human Kinetics, unless otherwise specified; photo on p. 1 © Comstock; photo on p. 61 © Monkey Business/fotolia.com; **Photo Asset Manager:** Laura Fitch; **Visual Production Assistant:** Joyce Brumfield; **Photo Production Manager:** Jason Allen; **Art Manager:** Kelly Hendren; **Associate Art Manager:** Alan L. Wilborn; **Illustrator:** Keri Evans, unless otherwise specified; **Printer:** Versa Press

Printed in the United States of America   10   9   8   7   6   5   4   3   2   1

The paper in this book is certified under a sustainable forestry program.

Human Kinetics
Web site: www.HumanKinetics.com

United States: Human Kinetics, P.O. Box 5076, Champaign, IL 61825-5076
800-747-4457
e-mail: humank@hkusa.com

Canada: Human Kinetics, 475 Devonshire Road Unit 100, Windsor, ON N8Y 2L5
800-465-7301 (in Canada only)
e-mail: info@hkcanada.com

Europe: Human Kinetics, 107 Bradford Road, Stanningley, Leeds LS28 6AT, United Kingdom
+44 (0) 113 255 5665
e-mail: hk@hkeurope.com

Australia: Human Kinetics, 57A Price Avenue, Lower Mitcham, South Australia 5062
08 8372 0999
e-mail: info@hkaustralia.com

New Zealand: Human Kinetics, P.O. Box 80, Torrens Park, South Australia 5062
0800 222 062
e-mail: info@hknewzealand.com

E4965

CONTENTS

Preface   v

Acknowledgments   vii

PART

I

GETTING STARTED
1

Program Introduction **3**

Implementing the Program **15**

PART

II

WELLNESS WEEK
PLANS
25

Planning for Wellness Week 1 . . . . **27**

Planning for Wellness Week 2 . . . . **37**

Planning for Wellness Week 3 . . . . **45**

Planning for Wellness Week 4 . . . . **53**

PART

III

PROGRAM FOUNDATIONS
61

Links With Academic Achievement. 63

Educational and Scientific Foundations 67

The Obesity Epidemic 75

Appendix A: Celebration Activities   79

Appendix B: Program Assessments   92

Appendix C: Program Themes, Routines, and Messages   104

Appendix D: NASPE Standards   117

References and Suggested Resources   122

About the Authors   124

DVD User Instructions   126

PREFACE

Fitness for Life: Elementary School is a unique program that focuses attention on schoolwide wellness during four weeks of the school year. A primary objective of the program is to help schools incorporate coordinated activities that will enable them to meet national standards and guidelines for physical activity and nutrition as part of their school wellness policy. The program promotes healthy lifestyles in physical education and classrooms as well as in the entire school and community. Featured components of healthy lifestyles are sound nutrition and regular physical activity. The program is designed specifically for elementary school students and provides lesson plans for physical education, physical activities for the classroom (including video-led routines and afternoon activity breaks), and whole-school events and activities. The program is designed to be easy to use, engaging, and fun for teachers and students. More complete details are included in part I of this book.

Fitness for Life: Elementary School is the result of a team effort. Scott Wikgren, director of the Health, Physical Education, Recreation, and Dance division of Human Kinetics, was the driving force behind this project. He was responsible for bringing the successful and award-winning **Fitness for Life: High School** program to Human Kinetics and also was the driving force behind the award-winning **Fitness for Life: Middle School** program. With Scott's assistance, an author team and a team of expert consultants were assembled. Together, Scott and I chose Guy Le Masurier, Dolly Lambdin, and Meg Greiner as coauthors for the project. Ellen Abbadessa and Jeff Walkuski were chosen as consulting authors. Guy contributes youthful enthusiasm, an excellent ability to put words on paper in a meaningful way, and a practical understanding of the needs of school-age youth. Dolly, former President of the National Association for Sport and Physical Education (NASPE) and recipient of the

University of Texas' Massey Award for Excellence in Teacher Education, also brings years of practical experience working with both students and teachers, an understanding of pedagogical principles and curriculum planning, and sound leadership. Meg has been honored as a NASPE Elementary Physical Educator of the Year, Disney Outstanding Specialist Teacher, and a *USA Today* All-Star Teacher. She has years of practical experience and is known for her innovative methods of promoting physical activity for all children. Ellen, an elementary physical education teacher and supervisor, helped with all aspects of the program but particularly with the teacher resources. Jeff, known for his years as a professor of physical education pedagogy, also contributed to all aspects of the program but primarily contributed to the afternoon activities in the classroom guides and related teacher information in each classroom lesson.

Other consultants who contributed to the project are listed on the acknowledgments page (p. vii). The consultants provided field testing, critiques of activities and book content, and suggestions for revisions and improvement. Special thanks go out to Linda Coyle, the social studies, physical education, and health specialist for the Paradise Valley, Arizona, schools. We also thank her excellent physical education advisory committee members for their input at all stages of program development and for their help in field testing the program. Many of the **Fitness for Life** instructors who participate in a program jointly sponsored by Physical Best and Human Kinetics also provided input.

Finally, I (and my coauthors) cannot say enough about the excellent work done by our editors, Ray Vallese and Derek Campbell, and our video and audio production partners, Doug Fink, Chris Johns, and Roger Francisco. In many ways Ray was really a coauthor of the program; not only did he do excellent development work and project coordination, but he also contributed many ideas and excellent content. Derek contributed in many similar ways. Both editors worked long hours and were diligent far beyond the call of duty. Doug and Chris were the creative minds behind the video productions and deserve Oscars for their work. Roger is the real pro who provided us with the music and other audio resources necessary for making the project a success. We cannot thank these people enough for their hard work and attention to detail. We would also like to thank all of the other people at Human Kinetics who contributed to this team effort.

Charles B. "Chuck" Corbin

ACKNOWLEDGMENTS

Many people played a role in the development of **Fitness for Life: Elementary School**. The following list credits the people who made this program possible. As noted in the preface, many others at Human Kinetics also contributed, and we acknowledge them all.

Video (Human Kinetics)

- Doug Fink, producer/director
- Roger Francisco, audio director
- Gregg Henness, camera operator/production assistant/teleprompter operator/Avid editor/DVD programmer
- Bill Yauch, camera operator
- Dan Walker, location audio
- Mark Herman, Avid editor/DVD programmer
- Chris Clark, Avid editor
- Sean Roosevelt, computer graphics art designer
- Stuart Cartwright, computer graphics art designer
- Amy Rose, production coordinator
- Chris Johns, scripts

Video Production (Camera Originals, Oak Brook, Illinois)

- Caren Cosby, producer/assistant director
- David Pierro, director of photography
- Dave Cosby, camera operator
- Tom McCosky, camera operator
- Ian Vacek, camera assistant
- Mark Markley, lighting
- Peter Horowitz, grip
- E.J. Huntemann, grip
- Dave Jack, audio technician
- Jackie Florczak, makeup/wardrobe
- Sarah Murphy, production coordinator
- Lauryn Kardatzke, production assistant

- Casey Lock, production assistant
- Kim Williams, O'Connor Casting

Video Hosts (K-2)

- David Goodloe
- Britni Tozzi

Video Hosts (3-6)

- Akula Lyman
- Laura Ball

Video Messages (authors)

- Chuck Corbin
- Guy Le Masurier
- Dolly Lambdin
- Meg Greiner
- Ellen Abbadessa (contributor)
- Jodi Le Masurier (contributor)

Audio/Music (Human Kinetics)

- Roger Francisco

Music Lyrics

- Chuck Corbin

Lyrics Advisors

- Cathie Corbin
- Dave Corbin
- Kris Youngkin
- Joan Milligan
- Dolly Lambdin

All About Dance Studio

- Jessica Goldman

Dance Consultants

- Josie Metal-Corbin
- Cathie Corbin
- Katie Corbin

- Julia Corbin
- Molly Corbin
- Suzi Corbin
- Joan Milligan

Performers (K-2)

- Christopher Chu
- Rohan Jain
- Carlton Jenkins
- Alex Rich
- Hayden Whitley
- Vincent Wilkinson
- Princess Jenkins
- Olivia Klein
- Brooke Kolker
- Claire Seymour
- Mollie Smithson
- Emma Weiss
- Chloe Zoller

Performers (3-6)

- Krystal Anderson
- Nair Banks
- Allie Bensinger
- Lauren Borg
- Caroline Chu
- Courtney Cosby
- Emily Schwartz
- Ashlyn Wiebe
- Aram Wilkinson
- Benjie Barclay
- Travis Little
- Kyle Birnbaum
- Nick Lucero
- Robert Banks

Performers (Guide for Wellness Coordinators DVD)

- Mollee Carter
- Ana Martinez
- Jose Quiroz

- Heaven Reed
- Rufina Reutov
- Rolando Sifuentez

Teacher Consultants

Paradise Valley, Arizona

- Linda Coyle, social studies, physical education & health, curriculum specialist
- Jay Thomas, Pinnacle High School
- Tonya Schwailler, Horizon High School
- Tammy Butler, Mountain Trail Middle School
- Craig Vogenson, Explorer Middle School
- Michael Wooldridge, Village Vista Elementary School
- Michele Popa, Desert Springs Elementary School
- Becki Griffen, Copper Canyon Elementary School
- George Mang, Pinnacle Peak Elementary School
- Susie Etchenbarren, PVUSD Adaptive Physical Education

Austin, Texas

- Laura Mikulencak, Pillow Elementary School
- Courtney Perry, Barton Hills Elementary School
- Tammy Arredondo, Graham Elementary School

Phoenix, Arizona

- Suzi Corbin

Contributing Authors

- Ellen Abbadessa
- Jeff Walkuski

Physical Best Authors

- Laura Borsdorf
- Lois Boeyink
- NASPE in association with AAHPERD

Dance Credits

- Harvest Time: movements adapted, with permission, from a video of a traditional African harvest dance (Djole) by Charles Ahovissi.

- Tinikling: movements adapted from Corbin, C.B. (1969), *Becoming physically educated in the elementary school,* Philadelphia: Lea & Febiger, used by permission of author and copyright owner, pages 323-329.

- Jumpnastics: movements adapted from Corbin, C.B. & Corbin, D.E. (1972), *Inexpensive equipment for games, play and physical activity,* Dubuque, IA: Brown, used by permission of authors and copyright owners, pages 49-50.

- Stomp and Balance: adapted from the Danish dance Seven Jumps as described by Corbin, C.B. (1969), *Becoming physically educated in the elementary school,* Philadelphia: Lea & Febiger, used by permission of author and copyright owner, pages 308-309, credit to RCA records, 1958 for original permission (now out of print).

- Hip Hop 5: adapted from a routine created by Mychal Taylor, Cecily Taylor, and Josie Metal-Corbin, used by permission.

- Keep on Clapping: adapted from a routine created by Mychal Taylor, Cecily Taylor, and Josie Metal-Corbin, used by permission.

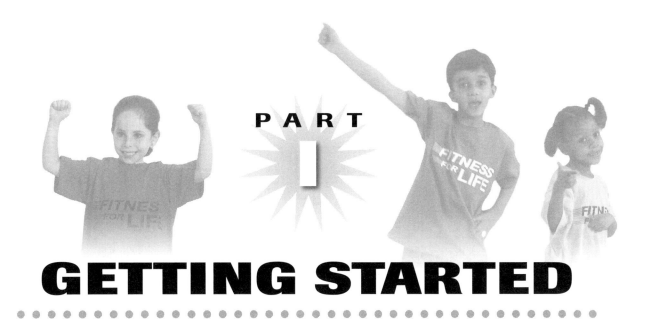

P A R T

I

GETTING STARTED

● ●

Part I of this guide provides a general introduction to the **Fitness for Life: Elementary School** program and a more detailed
section on implementing the program.

  • **Program Introduction** (page 3): This
    section introduces the **Fitness for Life:
    Elementary School** program. It provides
    a rationale for the program, including
    descriptions of the program foundations.
    The various program components and
    responsibilities are also described.

  • **Implementing the Program** (page 15):
    This section provides a detailed list of
    duties of the wellness coordinator. The
    resources available to the coordinator are
    also described. This section also includes
    an Executive Summary (page 17) that dis-
    tills the rationale and main components of
    the **Fitness for Life: Elementary School**
    program into a single page.

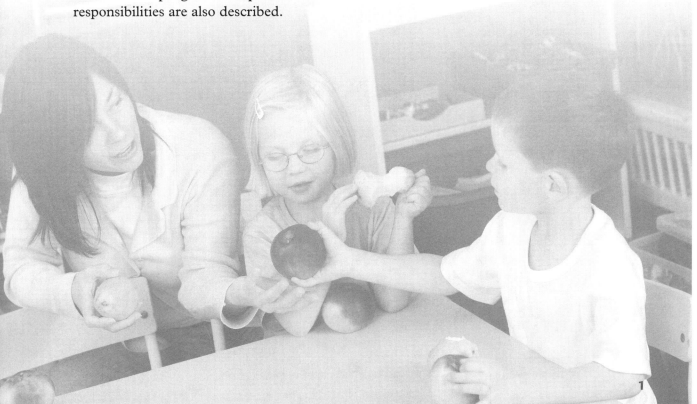

PROGRAM INTRODUCTION

Fitness for Life Elementary School

Fitness for Life: Elementary School (**FFL: Elementary**) is a unique program that focuses on schoolwide wellness. It provides curriculum materials for the classroom and physical education classes, as well as schoolwide activities and take-home information that promote healthy lifestyles in the school and the community. The healthy lifestyles components feature sound nutrition and regular physical activity. The program is designed specifically for elementary school students and involves the entire school, including teachers, administrators, and staff.

Program Rationale

Every school that receives federal school lunch program money must develop and carry out a school wellness policy. **FFL: Elementary** helps schools carry out a wellness plan. It supple-

ments other school programs, such as physical education, health curricula, and school cafeteria programs. It provides a focal point for healthy lifestyle promotion on a schoolwide basis. Some important outcomes of **FFL: Elementary** include the following:

- **Helping children meet national physical activity guidelines**. National physical activity guidelines call for 60 minutes of physical activity each day for every child. Many youth do not get the recommended amount of activity (United States Department of Health and Human Services [USDHHS], 2008). **FFL: Elementary** helps students meet the guidelines and is especially important to children whose daily activity outside of school is low.

- **Helping children avoid becoming overweight or obese**. Childhood obesity has tripled since the 1980s. Today, more

Some of the information provided in this section is similar to information provided in the introduction to the classroom guides and the *Physical Education Lesson Plans*. This overlap is intentional. Not all teachers read the same books, and it is important for everyone to get similar information. This guide includes more detail about the **Fitness for Life: Elementary School** program and its educational foundations than the other guides. For this reason, wellness coordinators may want to lend this guide to classroom teachers, physical education teachers, and others who want more information about the program.

than 15 percent of children are classified as obese, and an additional 15 percent or more are classified as overweight (Ogden et al., 2008). Regular physical activity and sound nutrition can contribute significantly to solving the problem.

- **Helping children avoid long periods of inactivity**. National guidelines indicate that children should not be inactive for long periods of time. We often condemn television watching and excessive use of computer games by children because they promote inactivity, yet schools often do the same thing—keep children inactive for long periods of time. Providing activity breaks and teaching children about physical activity and nutrition are good educational policies.

- **Helping children eat well**. Reinforcing sound nutrition in **FFL: Elementary** programs can help children improve nutrition

WHAT IS WELLNESS?

The **Fitness for Life: Elementary School** program focuses on wellness for school children. It includes Wellness Week activities that can be used to implement wellness policy as mandated by federal law. To implement an effective wellness program, it is helpful to have a clear understanding of the meaning of the word *wellness.* Many years ago, the World Health Organization defined health as being more than absence of disease (WHO, 1947). It was agreed that wellness, not just sickness, should be included in a definition of good health. The characteristics of wellness include the following:

* Wellness is part of good health.
* Wellness is a state of being exemplified by quality of life and a sense of well-being. Examples of quality of life and a sense of well-being from the health goals for our nation include the ability to perform activities of daily life without restriction, happiness, satisfaction with our lives, self-esteem, and a positive outlook on life.
* Wellness is considered the positive component of good health (more than freedom from illness).

* Health and its positive component (wellness) are integrated; each interacts with the other, and if one is influenced, both are influenced.
* Both health and wellness are multidimensional. The most commonly described dimensions are physical, social, intellectual, emotional (mental), and spiritual.

Two healthy lifestyles prominent in **FFL: Elementary** are regular physical activity and sound nutrition. These two lifestyles have been shown to have a positive impact on wellness and to reduce the risk of chronic diseases. Especially important is the fact that regular physical activity and sound nutrition are factors in life over which people have control. For this reason, these two behaviors are considered to be high-priority lifestyles. They can be changed with the help of educators and sound educational programs such as **FFL: Elementary.** Those who adopt healthy lifestyles will have improved health and wellness. Wellness programs typically include an emphasis on physical activity and nutrition because of their known benefits to personal wellness.

Adapted from Corbin, C.B., & Pangrazi, R.P. 2001. Toward a uniform definition of wellness: A commentary. *President's Council on Physical Fitness and Sports Research Digest, 3*(15), 1-8. Available at www.fitness.gov/publications/digests/pcpfs_research_digs.html.

habits, help prevent obesity, and improve general health.

- **Enhancing academic achievement**. Recent evidence clearly shows that time taken during the school day to involve children in physical activity does not decrease academic learning. In fact, there is ample evidence that physical activity breaks during the day enhance academic learning (Hillman et al., 2009a; Hillman et al., 2009b; Le Masurier & Corbin, 2006; Ratey, 2008; Smith & Lounsbery, 2009).

- **Stimulating cognitive function.** Benefits of regular physical activity include improved blood flow and vascular supply to the brain and increased production of brain-derived neurotrophic factor (BDNF) that supports neural connections (Ratey, 2008).

- **Helping your school fulfill its wellness plan**. All schools receiving federal funding for school meal programs must have a policy and comply with it (Le Masurier & Corbin, 2006). Taking the time to include **FFL: Elementary** in your program will help you and your school meet the school wellness policy requirement.

Program Organization

Fitness for Life: Elementary School is constructed to focus attention on physical activity and nutrition during four weeks of the school year. One week in every nine weeks of school is designated as Wellness Week. During each Wellness Week, the entire school focuses on wellness, emphasizing sound nutrition and regular physical activity. The exact dates of each Wellness Week are determined by the school staff. A wellness coordinator will be chosen to help coordinate the week's activities. In many cases, the physical education teacher will serve as wellness coordinator; however, the coordinator could be a classroom teacher, a nurse, a school staff member, or even a parent.

You may find the **FFL: Elementary** format so engaging and helpful that you want to include the activities every week, which would be great. But the basic program involves classroom

activities during one week of every nine weeks of school.

Each Wellness Week has two themes: one for physical activity and one for nutrition. Daily wellness messages are emphasized during Wellness Week. Table 1.1 illustrates the themes and basic messages for each Wellness Week; appendix C provides more detailed versions of these messages. Special schoolwide nutrition activities are planned every Wednesday (Eat Well Wednesday), and schoolwide physical activities are planned every Friday (Get Fit Friday). If you are not the wellness coordinator, you may be called upon to assist with these activities.

Wellness Coordinator

Because **FFL: Elementary** is a total school program, it must have a leader to be effective. Each school should select a wellness coordinator (who will use this guide) to oversee and direct program activities for each of the four Wellness Weeks during the school year, including the Eat Well Wednesday and Get Fit Friday activities. Of course, the coordinator may delegate responsibilities to other teachers and staff members in the school. One of the first duties of the coordinator is to have a meeting with school staff to explain **FFL: Elementary**. The DVD-ROM included with this guide includes resources to help the coordinator present the program to school staff.

See page 15 for a more detailed description of the duties of the wellness coordinator.

Program Package

There are nine books in the **FFL: Elementary** program package (see figure 1.1). Each book is color coded to facilitate easy identification and comes with one or more disks of videos and resources. The wellness coordinator will distribute the books to the appropriate school staff members. Schools that have more than one teacher for a specific grade level will need to share resources or purchase additional classroom guides.

The *Guide for Wellness Coordinators* (the book you are holding) includes a DVD with TEAM Time activity videos, a PowerPoint presentation, and many other resources, including signs,

Table 1.1 Themes and Messages for Each Wellness Week

Wellness Week	Activity theme	Nutrition theme	Daily messages for K-2	Daily messages for 3-5	Daily messages for 6
Week 1 (held in fall, or during the first 9 weeks of the school year)	Moderate physical activity	Fruits and vegetables	1: Be active every day. 2: Keep on trying. 3: Fitness foods 4: Play safely. 5: I can, you can, we all can.	1: 60 minutes every day 2: The more you practice, the better you get. 3: Eat 5 a day. 4: Start with safety. 5: Fun for me, fun for you, fun for all.	1: There are lots of fun physical activities. 2: Practice builds skills. 3: You are what you eat. 4: Safety is key for staying healthy. 5: I can!
Week 2 (held in fall/winter, or during the second 9 weeks of the school year)	Vigorous physical activity (vigorous aerobics, sports, and recreation)	Grains and high-calorie foods	1: Get your body moving! 2: Get better with practice. 3: Foods with fats 4: Exercise your heart. 5: Never, ever give up!	1: Play for a good day. 2: Build skills, have more fun. 3: Avoid empty calories. 4: Aerobic activity every day 5: Show respect.	1: Active all day 2: Start with the basics. 3: High-calorie foods 4: Heartbeats for health 5: Self-respect
Week 3 (held in winter/spring, or during the third 9 weeks of the school year)	Muscle fitness and flexibility exercises	Protein	1: Get your muscles ready. 2: Move your body. 3: Food for strong bones and muscles 4: You only have one body; make it fit! 5: If it is to be, it's up to me.	1: Take care of your muscles. 2: Practice for fitness. 3: Protein power 4: Be specific; look terrific. 5: Don't be a character—have character.	1: There is no "I" in "team". 2: Feedback to improve 3: Protein is important. 4: You get what you train for. 5: Rules rule!
Week 4 (held in spring, or during the fourth 9 weeks of the school year)	Integration (energy balance)	Energy balance	1: Get off your seat and move your feet. 2: Play lots, learn lots. 3: Healthy food helps us move. 4: Be water wise. 5: Plan to get better.	1: Brain and body exercise 2: Combine skills just for the fun of it. 3: Balance energy in (food) with energy out (exercise). 4: Water, water, before I get hotter! 5: Personal fitness starts with you.	1: Build a healthy body; build a healthy mind. 2: One step at a time 3: Balance calories. 4: Hit the water. 5: SMART goals

This table presents the overall nutrition theme for each Wellness Week; each grade range has a more specific variation of that theme. For example, the K-2 nutrition theme for Wellness Week 1 is "Fruits and vegetables (fitness foods)."

newsletters, assessments, and more. The cover and spine of this guide are red.

There are seven classroom guides, one for each grade from K to 6. The covers and spines change color based on the grade grouping: yellow and orange for the K-2 guides, shades of purple for the 3-5 books, and blue for the grade 6 book. Each guide presents classroom lesson plans for all five days of each Wellness Week. Each guide also includes a DVD that contains instructional videos and activity videos to use during the daily classroom activity breaks. In addition, each DVD contains signs, worksheets, and other printable resources for use by classroom teachers.

The *Physical Education Lesson Plans* book provides complete lesson plans for physical education classes for grades K-2 and grades 3-6. The cover and spine of this book are green. The book includes:

- a DVD with the instructional videos for the classroom routines,
- a DVD with selected daily videos from the classroom routines,
- a resources CD-ROM with signs, activity cards, and other printable resources, and
- a music CD with music and tracks for fitness testing for use with physical education lessons.

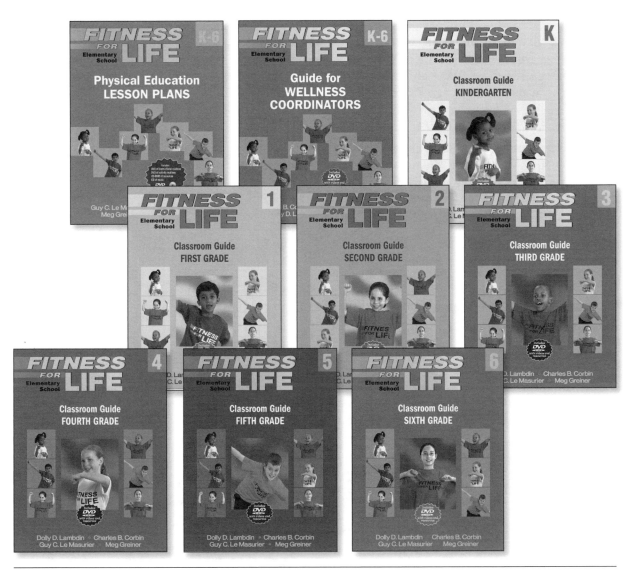

Figure 1.1   There are nine color-coded guides, one for each classroom teacher (grades K-6), one for the physical education teacher, and one for the wellness coordinator.

Program Components

The components of Wellness Week include the following:

- **Classroom activity breaks using video routines** created especially for **FFL: Elementary**. The lesson plans for using these routines are provided in the classroom guide for each grade, and the routines are included on the DVD in each guide.

- **Classroom activity breaks using additional activities** that reinforce academic concepts in subjects such as math, science, and language arts. Plans for these breaks are included in the classroom guide for each grade.

- **Physical education lesson plans**, including one warm-up lesson for use the week before each Wellness Week and three lesson plans for use during each Wellness Week. These lesson plans are provided in the *Physical Education Lesson Plans* book.

- **Conceptual learning discussions** related to wellness (focusing on nutrition and physical activity) using messages on the DVD video routines. These are done in the classroom and in physical education class.

- **Signs** for the classroom, the gym, the cafeteria, and school bulletin boards promoting sound nutrition and regular physical activity. These are provided among the resource materials for each book.

- **Chants** to reinforce the major messages of each lesson.

- **Eat Well Wednesdays** that feature schoolwide nutrition activities (including those for the cafeteria). The general nutrition themes for each Wellness Week are shown in table 1.1, and the special schoolwide nutrition activities are described later in this guide. The wellness coordinator works with the cafeteria staff to conduct the activities.

- **Get Fit Fridays** that feature schoolwide physical activities called TEAM Time activities; TEAM stands for "Together Everyone Achieves More." The TEAM Time activities are organized by the wellness coordina-

tor with the help of all school staff. More details are provided later in this guide.

- **Other schoolwide events** (celebration activities) promoting sound nutrition and regular physical activity. These events, described in appendix A, are coordinated by the wellness coordinator with the help of all school staff.

- **Newsletters** for distribution to families during Wellness Week. It is recommended that the wellness coordinator and administrative staff print these newsletters and give them to teachers to distribute to families. However, they can also be printed by classroom teachers or the physical education teacher, and they can be sent to families by e-mail. Newsletters are provided among the resource materials for each book and can be customized to suit local needs.

- **Worksheets** for use in promoting sound nutrition and physical activity. Worksheets are used in the classroom and in physical education, and they are provided among the resource materials for each book.

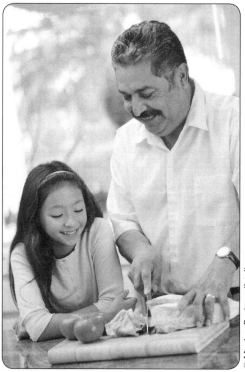

Eating well is the focus of Eat Well Wednesday activities.

- **FFL: Elementary Web site.** A Web site dedicated to the program is available at www.fitnessforlife.org. This site provides information for teachers, students, and parents.

Program Responsibilities

Responsibilities for different members of the school staff are listed below. Duties for the wellness coordinator are listed first.

Wellness Coordinator

- Conducts a faculty–staff meeting to explain Wellness Week (uses the PowerPoint® presentation and the Executive Summary provided on the DVD).
- Coordinates Wellness Week activities.
- Oversees schoolwide events such as Eat Well Wednesday and Get Fit Friday activities.
- Distributes materials to teachers and staff (e.g., Wellness Week newsletters, plans for Wellness Week schoolwide events).
- Provides in-service as necessary.
- See page 15 for a more detailed description of the duties of the wellness coordinator.

Physical Education Teacher

- Teaches the warm-up lesson the week before each Wellness Week. This includes teaching the video routine to be performed in the classroom during Wellness Week.
- Teaches lessons during Wellness Week.
- Posts Wellness Week signs in the gym or multipurpose room.
- Assists with schoolwide events planned by wellness coordinator (e.g., Eat Well Wednesday, Get Fit Friday, celebration activities).
- May serve as the wellness coordinator—if so, performs duties listed previously. This guide provides more details. In addition, the physical education teacher may wish to obtain an excellent article titled "Preparing physical educators

for the role of physical activity director" (Beighle et al., 2009), which can help them or anyone who serves as wellness coordinator.

Classroom Teacher

- Conducts activity breaks in the classroom using video routines on the DVD included with each classroom guide.
- Conducts discussions about wellness messages included on the videos.
- Conducts integrated activities in math, science, and other academic areas as outlined in the lesson plans in the classroom guides.
- Conducts the classroom discussion for Eat Well Wednesday.
- Posts the Wellness Week signs (printed from the classroom guide DVD) in the classroom.
- May send home the Wellness Week newsletter (provided by the wellness coordinator or printed from the classroom guide DVD).
- Uses classroom worksheets as appropriate (printed from the classroom guide DVD).
- Assists with schoolwide events planned by the wellness coordinator (e.g., Eat Well Wednesday, Get Fit Friday, celebration activities).

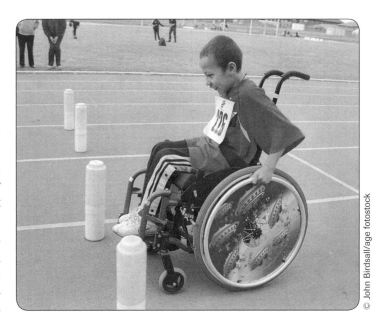

© John Birdsall/age fotostock

Wellness Week activities help all students to be active.

School Principal

- Appoints or aids in selection of the wellness coordinator.

- Provides enthusiastic support for the **FFL: Elementary** program.

- Participates in schoolwide Wellness Week activities.

Art Teacher

- Works with the wellness coordinator and classroom teachers to promote wellness, physical activity, and nutrition during each Wellness Week.

- Has students create art related to wellness for posting on school walls (or as part of a wellness art show).

Music Teacher

- Works with classroom and physical education teachers to promote wellness during Wellness Week.

- Helps students learn songs from the video routines (on the classroom guide DVDs) to be performed in the classroom.

- Helps students learn the words to "Colors," the song used in the TEAM Time 2: Big Kids Lead activity (see page 42 for more details).

Librarian or Computer Teacher

- Identifies books on wellness, nutrition, and physical activity and encourages students to read them during Wellness Week.

- Supports computer activities related to Wellness Week (e.g., MyPyramid Tracker, Activitygram).

Nutrition Staff

- Conducts schoolwide nutrition activities on Eat Well Wednesday.

- Posts Wellness Week nutrition signs in school and cafeteria.

Other Staff

- Assists the wellness coordinator with schoolwide events.

- Assists in printing and posting Wellness Week signs.

Parents

- Help with schoolwide events.

- Encourage children to be active and eat well, especially during Wellness Week.

Educational Foundations

Fitness for Life: Elementary School is based on sound educational foundations. Some of the key information that was considered in building

---

HELP TEACHERS FIND THE TIME FOR CLASSROOM ACTIVITIES

Classroom teachers have many subjects to cover during the school day. Some may feel that they do not have time for classroom physical activities during Wellness Week. Help these teachers understand that the time taken for Wellness Week activities will not only improve student health and fitness but will also contribute to achievement in the classroom and to better test performance (Hillman et al., 2009a; Hillman et al., 2009b; Le Masurier & Corbin, 2006; Ratey, 2008; Smith & Lounsbery, 2009). Taking just 1 to 3 minutes from each hour of the school day (or 1 to 3 minutes from five activities during the day) will provide the time needed for classroom Wellness Week activities. You can also remind teachers that Wellness Week occurs only four times a year.

the program is summarized in this section. More comprehensive coverage of the educational foundations for **FFL: Elementary** is available in part III of this guide.

Child Nutrition and WIC Reauthorization Act

In 2004, the United States Congress passed the Child Nutrition and Women, Infants and Children (WIC) Reauthorization Act (Public Law 108-265). As a result of the act, all states, school districts, and schools receiving funding for school lunch programs must have a policy (plan) designed to encourage total school wellness. Central to a sound wellness policy is the notion that the primary mission of schools is to promote optimal learning for all children, and this cannot be achieved if students are not fit, healthy, and well. **FFL: Elementary** helps schools meet key guidelines of the legislation and can help your school meet wellness planning guidelines. Action for Healthy Kids is a national group dedicated to promoting school wellness and has many online tools to help implement school wellness plans. For more information, log on to www.actionforhealthykids.org.

USDHHS National Physical Activity Guidelines for Children

In October of 2008, the U.S. Department of Health and Human Services (USDHHS) published national physical activity guidelines for children. These guidelines, as abstracted below, were used in developing the **FFL: Elementary** program. For more details, visit www.health.gov/paguidelines.

- Children should perform physical activity 60 minutes (or more) each day. Choose from either moderate (equal in intensity to brisk walking) or vigorous activity (activity that elevates heart rate).
- Children should perform vigorous activity at least 3 days per week.
- Children should perform stretching and muscle fitness activities that build muscles and bones at least 3 days per week.
- Activities should be age appropriate, enjoyable, and varied.

USDA National Nutrition Guidelines

Every five years, a committee of the U.S. Department of Agriculture (USDA) revises the national nutrition guidelines. A recent revision resulted in the development of MyPyramid (see figure 1.2). The nutrition component of the **FFL: Elementary** program relies heavily on information associated with MyPyramid for Kids. The steps on the side of MyPyramid for Kids represent the various forms of physical activity that are also depicted in the Physical Activity Pyramid for Kids (see figure 1.3). The USDA nutrition guidelines emphasize the importance of physical activity and sound nutrition in promoting health and wellness.

The DVD in this guide includes a color version of MyPyramid for Kids. The pyramid is provided as one of the general signs for use

EAT 5 TO 9 A DAY

To encourage consumption of a variety of fruits and vegetables, the **FFL: Elementary** program uses the simple "5 to 9 servings a day" message that is designed to help children meet national recommendations. For cooked vegetables, 1/2 cup equals one serving, and for leafy vegetables, 1 cup equals one serving. One medium apple, banana, or pear equals one fruit serving. The Centers for Disease Control and Prevention (CDC) uses the "Fruits & Veggies—More Matters" campaign to encourage more fruits and veggies in the diet. For more information, visit the following Web sites:

- ✳ www.fruitsandveggiesmatter.gov
- ✳ www.mypyramid.gov/pyramid/ fruits_counts.html
- ✳ www.mypyramid.gov/pyramid/ vegetables_counts.html

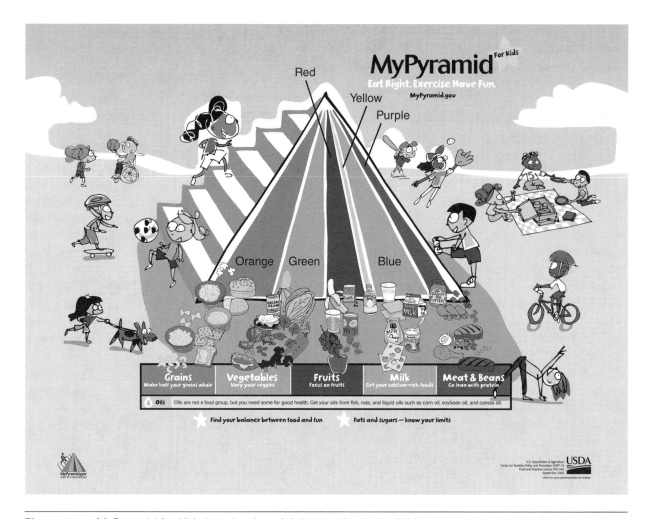

Figure 1.2   MyPyramid for Kids is a visual model designed to help children learn about each of the major food groups. MyPyramid is used extensively in the **FFL: Elementary** program. For more information, go to www.mypyramid.gov.

Adapted from U.S. Department of Agriculture.

during any Wellness Week (see page 19 for details about the general signs).

Physical Activity Pyramid for Kids

The Physical Activity Pyramid for Kids (see figure 1.3) illustrates the different types of physical activity that can be used to promote good health, fitness, and wellness. The basic pyramid is used in all **Fitness for Life** programs, but there is a special version just for young children; the upper-level programs use the Physical Activity Pyramid for Teens. The Physical Activity Pyramid for Kids helps children better understand the benefits of the different types of activity. As noted earlier, each of the four Wellness Weeks

focuses on a different type of physical activity from the pyramid.

The Physical Activity Pyramid for Kids has five colored steps that represent different types of activity.

- Moderate activity is represented by step 1 (orange). It includes activities equal to brisk walking, including active play for children. It is at the base of the pyramid because it is the most commonly performed activity and can be done regularly by all people.

- Step 2 (green) includes vigorous aerobics. Activities that are vigorous enough to elevate the heart rate in the heart rate

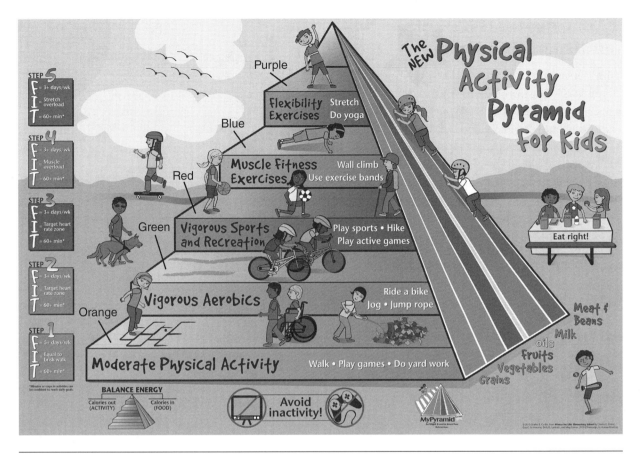

Figure 1.3   The Physical Activity Pyramid for Kids is a visual model designed to help children learn about the five major physical activity types.

©2010 Charles B. Corbin

target zone are considered to be vigorous aerobics. Jogging, biking at a relatively fast pace, and lap swimming are examples.

- Step 3 (red) includes vigorous sports and recreation such as tennis, soccer, and hiking. Only activities that elevate the heart rate sufficiently are considered to be vigorous in nature. Some sports and recreational activities such as bowling are classified as moderate (step 1).

- Step 4 (blue) includes exercises for muscle fitness. Climbing on a climbing structure, calisthenics such as push-ups or curl-ups, elastic band exercises, and stunts that require the use of arms and legs to move the body (e.g., crab walk) are examples of muscle fitness exercises.

- Step 5 (purple) includes flexibility exercises. Activities that require the muscles

to stretch beyond their normal length are called flexibility exercises. Examples are gymnastics stunts, yoga, and stretching calisthenics (e.g., sit and reach).

National guidelines for children recommend activity from all steps of the pyramid. Children need 60 minutes of activity daily from steps 1 to 3. Inactivity or sedentary living is shown below the pyramid. Extended periods of inactivity (e.g., watching TV, playing inactive computer games) should be avoided.

For more details on the Physical Activity Pyramid for Kids, see the educational foundations in part III of this guide. The DVD in this guide includes a color version of the pyramid. The pyramid is provided as one of the general signs for use during any Wellness Week (see page 19 for details about the general signs).

NASPE Physical Education Curriculum Standards

The National Association for Sport and Physical Education (NASPE) has developed standards for the physical education curriculum (NASPE, 2004). These standards have been used by 48 of the 50 states in developing state standards and physical education curricula. The NASPE standards define the content needed to help individuals develop the knowledge, skills, and confidence to enjoy a lifetime of healthy physical activity. The physical education lessons, the classroom lessons, and the schoolwide activities are based on NASPE standards. A complete description of the NASPE standards is included in appendix D.

Curriculum Standards for Other Academic Areas

Curriculum standards in other areas such as math were considered in developing **FFL: Elementary** lessons. For more information about these other standards, see part III of this guide or appendix B of the classroom guides.

Fitness for Life Philosophy

Fitness for Life: Elementary School is part of a comprehensive K-12 program. In addition to **FFL: Elementary**, there are **Fitness for Life** programs for middle school and high school (see www.fitnessforlife.org for details). All **Fitness for Life** programs are based on the

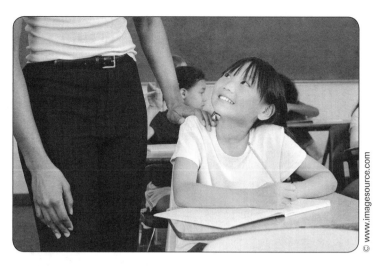

© www.imagesource.com

Fitness for Life: Elementary School helps students meet a variety of subject matter standards.

HELP philosophy. The first letters in four key words form the **HELP** acronym.

- **H**ealth. The program is designed to help elementary school students learn about health-related physical fitness and the benefits of healthy lifestyles, including regular physical activity and sound nutrition.
- **E**veryone. The program is designed for everyone (all elementary school students), not just those with special physical talents.
- **L**ifetime. The activities included in all **Fitness for Life** programs were chosen to get kids active now as well as build habits that will last a lifetime.
- **P**ersonal. All lessons are designed to help each student learn personally appropriate physical activity and nutrition information.

IMPLEMENTING THE PROGRAM

This section of the guide details the duties of the wellness coordinator. First, it explains how to present the **Fitness for Life: Elementary School** program to school staff so that they become familiar with the components and understand how everything works together. Next, it walks you through the eight steps to follow when planning each Wellness Week. These steps present a general overview of the planning process; part II of this guide (starting on page 25) provides the specific details on planning for weeks 1, 2, 3, and 4.

The DVD in this guide contains videos and resources for use during the four Wellness Weeks. When you insert the disk in a DVD player, the screen will display a menu of videos. When you access the disk through your computer's DVD-ROM drive, you will see five folders of resources: General, Wellness Week 1, Wellness Week 2, Wellness Week 3, and Wellness Week 4. This section explains how to use the videos and resources when implementing the program. (For technical details on inserting and opening the DVD, see page 126.)

Throughout this guide, references to printable resources are accompanied by an icon and folder path to remind you of where to find the resources on the DVD. For example, when the text asks you to send out the newsletter for Wellness Week 1, the following shows you where to find the file:

 Wellness Week 1 → Newsletter

Because the printable resources on the DVD are intended to be engaging, most are presented in color, but they will print normally to black-and-white printers as well. If you have a color printer but wish to conserve your color ink, you can print the resources in grayscale. For details on how to do this, check your printer's instruction manual, or click the Help or Properties button in your Print window.

All contents of the DVD are intended for use only by instructors and agencies that have purchased this guide. The reproduction of the contents of the DVD is otherwise forbidden according to the terms stated on the copyright page of this guide.

Presenting to School Staff

Early in the school year, after the rush of the first few weeks of school, the wellness coordinator will make a presentation to the school staff to inform them of the details of the **Fitness for Life: Elementary School** program and the four Wellness Weeks. The presentation can be made in a regular staff meeting or at a special meeting specifically called to introduce the program. The presentation (with time for questions) should take about 30 minutes.

The DVD includes several resources to help you make the presentation. First, you can use the PowerPoint slide show as the basis for the presentation, customizing the slides to suit your school's

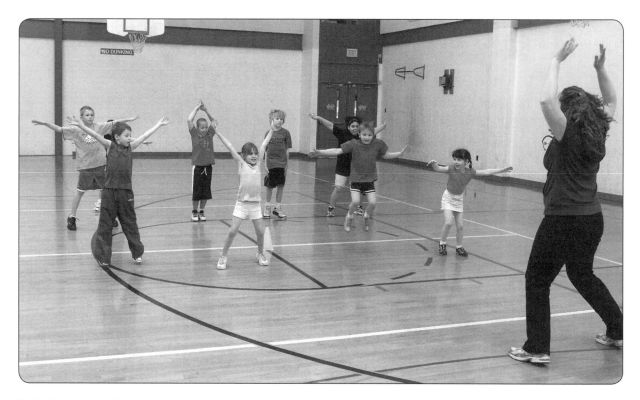

Schoolwide activities are featured each Wellness Week.

particular needs. Second, you can print the Executive Summary and distribute a copy to each staff member; the Executive Summary also appears on page 17 of this guide. Third, you can share the information in the *Model Guidelines for Health and Wellness* booklet (included in PDF format on the DVD), which explains how to develop school wellness policies to meet the requirements of the Child Nutrition and WIC Reauthorization Act.

 General → Planning

> Program Overview
>
> Executive Summary
>
> Model Guidelines

In addition, the DVD contains a video of a behind-the-scenes interview with Chuck Corbin, senior author of **Fitness for Life,** in which he discusses the development and objectives of the elementary program. You can play this interview during your meeting.

During the meeting, consult with the staff about possible dates for scheduling each Wellness Week. Work with school administrators, using input from staff, to determine the exact dates for each Wellness Week. Consider the following factors:

- Schedule one Wellness Week each 9 weeks.
- Consider holidays; try to schedule a week that has 5 days of school.
- Consider other schoolwide activities and avoid scheduling during other events.
- Avoid the first few weeks of school; allow time to get organized.
- Avoid periods when school testing is being conducted.

Key points for the presentation:

- Overview of **FFL: Elementary** program
- Overview of Wellness Week organization (one per 9 weeks of school)
- Reasons for Wellness Week
- Discussion of the school's wellness policy
- Roles for various staff members

A special **FFL: Elementary** Web site is available at www.fitnessforlife.org. If Web access is available, log onto the Web site, and show it to the school staff. Special sections are available for

EXECUTIVE SUMMARY

What Is Fitness for Life: Elementary School?

Fitness for Life: Elementary School (FFL: Elementary) is a program designed to promote wellness, physical activity, sound nutrition, and healthy lifestyles throughout the entire school.

Why Should I Do the Program?

Some of the principal benefits of **FFL: Elementary** are as follows:

* Helps your students meet national physical activity guidelines.
* Helps your school implement a wellness policy as required by law.
* Helps prevent childhood obesity by teaching about expending calories and limiting caloric intake.
* Helps build youth fitness.
* Helps children eat a healthy diet and meet national nutrition goals.
* Promotes academic achievement.
* Stimulates activity that increases blood flow to the brain.

What Are the Basic Components of the Program?

FFL: Elementary is a schoolwide wellness program that requires participation by all school employees and students. Once every nine weeks, the entire school conducts a Wellness Week (four each year). Major activities of each Wellness Week include the following:

* **Classroom activity breaks** that use teacher-friendly DVD videos and lesson plans
* **Physical education activities** that use provided lesson plans

* **Schoolwide special events** with plans for Eat Well Wednesday (a day of nutrition activities), Get Fit Friday (a day of TEAM Time physical activities), and celebration activities
* **School signs** promoting wellness to be posted throughout the school
* **Educational video messages** that teach children about wellness, sound nutrition, and physical activity
* **Worksheets** to reinforce learning about sound nutrition and physical activity
* **Newsletters** to help families get involved in Wellness Week
* A **Web site** to help students and families learn more about important wellness concepts

How Do I Find Time for the Program?

Time is at a premium in elementary school, and there are many educational goals to be met. So how can you find the time for **FFL: Elementary**? The program is conducted during four weeks each year so that a concentrated effort can be placed on wellness during these specific weeks. The classroom activity breaks can be done in 5 to 6 minutes. The total time for **FFL: Elementary** is 10 to 15 minutes per day. Research shows that time in physical activity can promote learning in the classroom, so the time is well spent. The breaks also promote fitness, health, and wellness. Taking 2 to 3 minutes from each hour of the school day will provide the time to conduct classroom activity breaks. The physical education lessons can be conducted in regular physical education classes and can be integrated into the regular physical education program.

teachers, students, and parents. Encourage those in attendance to explore the Web site. The newsletters provide Web site information to parents.

Planning Schoolwide Activities

The wellness coordinator helps all school staff implement the various Wellness Week activities. This section assumes that you are the wellness coordinator and walks you through eight steps to follow when planning each Wellness Week. You can print a checklist from the DVD (found in the following folder) that summarizes the steps to help you plan and conduct the week's activities.

 General → Planning

Step 1: Prepare Staff

Remind the physical education teacher (who could be you) to teach the Wellness Week lessons, using the *Physical Education Lesson Plans* book, the DVDs, the resources CD-ROM, and the music CD. The week before each Wellness Week, the physical education teacher should teach the video routine that will be used in the classroom (by classroom teachers) as a morning activity break during Wellness Week. The other physical education lesson plans will be taught during Wellness Week.

Remind the classroom teachers to prepare to teach their grade-specific lessons during Wellness Week. They should use the appropriate classroom guide to implement Wellness Week activities as described earlier. If students do not learn the classroom activity break routines from the physical education teacher, the classroom teachers can teach the routines instead using the instructional videos on the classroom guide DVDs. Once the students learn the routines, the classroom teachers will play one of the five video routines each day of the week.

Remind other staff of their responsibilities (as summarized starting on page 9).

Step 2: Distribute Newsletters

The **FFL: Elementary** program includes four newsletters, one for each Wellness Week. The newsletters are provided on the DVD in this guide, on the DVDs in the classroom guides, and on the resources CD-ROM in the *Physical Education Lesson Plans* book. This makes it easy for anyone—you, the classroom teachers, or the physical education teacher—to distribute the proper newsletter during each Wellness Week. If possible, try to use more than one form of distribution to increase the chances that you will reach everyone. Distribution options for the newsletters include:

- Office staff print the newsletters and distribute them to each classroom teacher for students to take home.
- Classroom teachers print and distribute the newsletters.
- You or the administrative staff sends the newsletters via e-mail. If your school has an e-mail distribution system, using this method saves time and paper.
- You or an administrative staff person posts the newsletter on your school Web page.

Most resources provided in the program are PDF files that you can print but not edit without special software. However, the newsletters are saved as Microsoft® Word® files so that you can customize them as needed. You can make each newsletter specific to your school or even to a particular class.

On the DVD in this guide, the newsletter for each Wellness Week is provided in the specific folder for that week.

 Wellness Week 1 → Newsletter

 Wellness Week 2 → Newsletter

 Wellness Week 3 → Newsletter

 Wellness Week 4 → Newsletter

Step 3: Post Signs

The DVD in this guide includes different types of signs that you can post throughout the school. These include the following:

- **General signs.** These signs can be printed during the first Wellness Week and reused during subsequent Wellness Weeks. The general signs include one for Eat Well Wednesday, one for Get Fit Friday, and one for TEAM Time.

- **Weekly signs**. These signs contain messages and information specific to each Wellness Week. Print them prior to the appropriate Wellness Week. All signs can be saved in folders for use in subsequent years.
- **Active playground signs**. These signs are designed to encourage activity on the playground. Step 4 explains how to use the signs.
- **Cafeteria signs**. These signs promote messages about good nutrition and can be posted in the cafeteria during each Wellness Week. Step 5 explains how to use the signs.
- **Table tent signs**. These folding signs are placed on cafeteria tables on each Eat Well Wednesday. Step 5 explains how to use the table tent signs.

The general signs and the specific Wellness Week signs are described in the following sections. The other signs are described in steps 4 and 5.

General Signs

These signs are general in nature and can be printed before the first Wellness Week and reused for all other Wellness Weeks. These signs are designed to be posted in school hallways and other common areas such as the school cafeteria. A list of general signs follows.

 General → General Signs

Blank horizontal

Blank vertical

G1: Fitness for Life: Elementary School

G2: Wellness Week

G3: Physical Activity Pyramid for Kids

G4: MyPyramid for Kids

G5: Eat Well Wednesday

G6: TEAM Time: Together Everyone Achieves More

G7: Get Fit Friday

G8: Healthy mind, healthy body, healthy heart . . . let's start!

G9: ABCs of Physical Activity

G10: ABCs of Nutrition

The signs are PDF files and can be printed but not edited (unless you have special software). For this reason, we have provided two blank signs that feature the **Fitness for Life: Elementary School** design but that have no message content. You can print these blank signs and customize them as desired, either by hand or by feeding the signs back through your printer.

The ABCs of Physical Activity file contains 27 signs, one for each letter of the alphabet and two signs for M (one about moderate activity and one about muscle fitness). The ABCs of Nutrition file contains 26 signs, one for each letter of the alphabet.

Suggested locations for posting the general signs include near the school entrance (G1 and G2), in the cafeteria (G4, G5, and G10), in the hallways (G5 and G7), in the school gym (G9), in other common areas (G1, G2, G3, G8, and G9), and in the location where the TEAM Time activity will be held (G6 and G7).

Weekly Signs

The specific Wellness Week signs are to be used during the appropriate Wellness Week. They can be posted in the hallways, on bulletin boards, and in the cafeteria when indicated. These signs feature themes and messages appropriate to each Wellness Week. If possible, have members of the office staff print the signs and post them. If this is not possible, you may want to have students help you print and post them before or after school. Consider laminating the signs so they last longer.

On the DVD in this guide, the specific signs for each Wellness Week are provided in the folder for that week. The signs for each week are saved together in one file so you can easily print them all at once.

 Wellness Week 1 → Weekly Signs

Physical Activity Pyramid: Moderate activity every day!

Green is for veggies, red is for fruits!

Whatever you love to play, get 60 minutes every day!

Move your muscles when you work and play!

The more you practice, the better you get!

Keep on trying. The more you try, the better you get!

Eat the rainbow way: every color, every day!

Play safely!

I can, you can, we all can work together!

Eat 5 a day, every day!

Start with safety! Finish with fun!

Fun for me, fun for all!

 Wellness Week 2 → Weekly Signs

Physical Activity Pyramid: Make some activity vigorous!

Orange is for grains!

Avoid empty calories!

A healthy body needs a healthy mind!

Get your body moving!

The more you practice, the better you play; practice, practice every day!

Making your heart beat fast helps your body last!

A healthy heart is a happy heart!

Exercising your heart daily really pays. Your heart will thank you in many ways!

Keep on going to get fit. Never give up! Never quit!

Play for a good day!

Activity + academics = a winning combination!

Build skills, have fun!

Make half your grains whole!

Get some aerobic activity every day!

Show respect—follow the golden rule!

To be fit, you must think FITT!

 Wellness Week 3 → Weekly Signs

Physical Activity Pyramid: Do exercise for muscle fitness and flexibility!

Blue is for milk; purple is for meat and beans!

A healthy mind needs a healthy body!

Before you play or perform, you need to get your muscles warm!

Music helps you move!

Protein power! Get strong, live long!

We have only one body. Let's make it fit!

If it is to be, it's up to me!

Building muscle requires skill and technique; strengthen your muscles three times per week!

Protein builds cells in muscles and brains; eat your protein foods and make big gains!

Be specific; look terrific!

Don't be a character; show your character!

Follow the rules and share the ball; demonstrate fairness, respect, and teamwork to all!

There is no "I" in "team"!

 Wellness Week 4 → Weekly Signs

Physical Activity Pyramid: Do activities from all the steps!

Eat all of the colors in the pyramid!

If you don't take care of your body, where will you live?

Get off your seat and move your feet!

Get up, get moving, and have some fun. It helps your brain when you get out and run!

Play lots, learn lots!

Play every day, sun or rain. Playing is good for your brain!

Healthy foods help us move! Choose your foods wisely!

Be water wise!

Be sun wise!

If you want to do better than before, make a plan to practice more!

When we play and train, we build our brains!

Combine skills to have some fun!

Energy in (the food we eat) – energy out (how much we move) = a healthy body

To play your best, drink water at every rest!

Personal fitness starts with me!

Step 4: Encourage Active Playgrounds

Even though students have free time on the playground, they are not necessarily active. The goal is to get all kids active when they are on the playground. You can help promote active playgrounds in the following ways.

- Print and post the active playground signs near doors to the playground. The goal is to get all children being active during free-play time.
- Ask staff members or teachers to make some activity equipment available during recess and lunch.
- Create an activity bin that has balls, jump ropes, and other equipment that can be wheeled out to activity areas.
- Teach some playground games that help children stay active during recess (see specific Wellness Week plans).
- Ask playground supervisors to verbally encourage active play.
- Create certain areas that are active zones where children must be active to play in these zones.

On the DVD in this guide, the active playground signs are found in the following folder. The signs are saved together in one file so you can easily print them all at once.

 General → Active Playground Signs

Active play area ahead: Get moving!

You have a green light! Get your body running!

No sitting, no standing! Get active, get moving!

Choose to be active!

Start your engine and get moving now!

Caution: Children moving ahead!

Don't sit, get fit!

Get off your seat and move your feet!

Step 5: Coordinate Eat Well Wednesday Activities

Eat Well Wednesday focuses on nutrition. The messages on all the video routines are devoted to nutrition. Classroom and physical education teachers should reinforce nutrition messages on each Eat Well Wednesday. School staff, including cafeteria staff, may want to reinforce the nutrition messages on these days.

There is a different nutrition theme for each Wellness Week, and that theme is reinforced during Eat Well Wednesday each week. The cafeteria signs for each Wellness Week reflect the messages for that week. The ABCs of Nutrition signs can be posted each week either in the cafeteria or in the hallways of the school. As noted in step 3, the general signs include an Eat Well Wednesday sign that can be posted in the cafeteria or hallway.

In addition, the DVD includes table tent signs that should be printed, folded, and placed on tables in the cafeteria on Eat Well Wednesdays. When each sign is folded, it forms a shape like a tent, with each side displaying the same nutrition message to students.

A variety of different nutrition special events are available for use on Eat Well Wednesdays. Some involve parents and some involve cafeteria staff. Details are included in the specific plans for each Wellness Week. In addition, because allergies can be a problem for some children, you may want to take some time to discuss food allergies on Eat Well Wednesdays.

Because the cafeteria signs are general and meant to be used during all Wellness Weeks, they are found in the following folder on the DVD. The signs are saved together in one file so you can easily print them all at once.

 General → Cafeteria Signs

Orange is for grains!

Green is for veggies!

Red is for fruits!

Blue is for milk products!

Purple is for meat and beans!

Yellow is for oils. Use them wisely!

Life is full of choices. Choose healthy foods!

Be wise. Eat well and exercise!

Food is fuel for learning and moving. Choose wisely!

Did you eat the rainbow way today?

Eat the rainbow way: every color, every day!

Did you eat your 5 to 9 today?

Make half your grains whole!

Protein power! Get strong, live long!

You are what you eat. Choose wisely!

Avoid empty calories!

The table tent signs, on the other hand, are not general. Each Wellness Week has two table tent signs that reinforce the nutrition message of that particular week. Thus, on the DVD, the table tent signs are found in the folder for each Wellness Week. The signs are saved together in one file so you can easily print them all at once.

 Wellness Week 1 → Tent Signs

Eat the rainbow way: every color, every day!

Fruits and vegetables: Eat 5 to 9 a day!

 Wellness Week 2 → Tent Signs

Eat breakfast: Make healthy choices!

Make half your grains whole!

 Wellness Week 3 → Tent Signs

Protein power! Get strong, live long!

Foods for strong bones and muscles

 Wellness Week 4 → Tent Signs

You are what you eat, from your head down to your feet!

Balance energy in (food) with energy out (activity)!

Step 6: Coordinate Get Fit Friday Activities

Get Fit Friday is devoted to special schoolwide physical activities. One schoolwide event is planned for each Wellness Week. The primary activity for the Get Fit Friday schoolwide activity is TEAM Time ("Together Everyone Achieves More"). TEAM Time activities are done in a 10-minute period before school. All children congregate in the school gym or multipurpose room (or outside if necessary). With the help of students, you will lead the TEAM Time activity described in the specific Wellness Week sections of this guide.

When you play the DVD in a DVD player, you can choose videos for four TEAM Time activities, one for each Wellness Week. Each activity has an instructional video that shows how a typical wellness coordinator might conduct the activity, plus one or more tracks that you can use when leading the activity in your school.

- TEAM Time 1: School Walk
  - Instructional
  - Music
- TEAM Time 2: Big Kids Lead
  - Instructional
  - Warm-up
  - Colors
  - Cool-down
- TEAM Time 3: Little Kids Lead
  - Instructional
  - We Get Fit
  - CYIM Fit
  - Wave It
- TEAM Time 4: Mid Kids Lead
  - Instructional
  - Warm-up
  - Hawaiian Surfing
  - Cool-down

The wellness coordinator in the instructional videos changes some of the activity details slightly to suit the needs of her school. For example, she uses the TEAM Time 1 activity as described, but she calls it the Wellness Walk instead of the School Walk. Feel free to make similar changes when you lead the TEAM Time activities to make them work best for you and your school.

The DVD also includes printable resources for use with the TEAM Time activities. These resources are found in the folder for each Wellness Week. The resources for each week are saved together in one file so you can easily print them all at once.

 Wellness Week 1 → TEAM Time

 Wellness Week 2 → TEAM Time

Wellness Week 3 → TEAM Time

 Wellness Week 4 → TEAM Time

Step 7: Coordinate Other Special Celebrations

You can conduct a variety of other special Wellness Week celebrations. It is recommended that one celebration activity be planned each Wellness Week so that four activities are conducted during the year. Below are brief descriptions of recommended celebration activities; see appendix A for more details. For some of the activities, resources are provided on the DVD.

 General → Celebrations

Brain Walk

The Brain Walk can be held before schoolwide or classroom tests or exams. Students walk through the school or on the playground before tests. The DVD includes a file of signs to use with this activity.

Family Fun Night

This is an organized school event in which students and families participate in a variety of physical activities that encourage them to play together. The DVD includes a flier that you can print and customize to promote Family Fun Night.

Fitness-a-Thon

Students participate in a variety of physical activities that are distributed around the play area. At each center, students play or practice a particular physical activity. The centers are monitored by teachers, who travel with their class from center to center.

Fun Run/Walk

Everyone walks or jogs simultaneously. Designate a course outside on the playground or field. Everyone joins in by jogging or walking around the area for a set amount of time. This activity can be organized by grade level, individual class, or physical education class. The DVD includes a certificate that you can award to students who participate in the Fun Run/Walk.

GYM Club

Start a GYM (Get Yourself Moving) club. Offer students access to the club before school, during recess, or after school, depending on your schedule. Activity examples include a jump rope club (which might include individual, double dutch, and long jump rope skills), a sport skills club (perhaps with basketball, volleyball, or soccer), a circus arts club (with stilts, juggling, flower sticks, diabolos, or unicycles), a dance club (with line, folk, square, modern, or hip-hop dances), and a muscle maniacs club (with organized games and activities that focus on muscle strength and endurance). The DVD includes a sample jump rope certificate that you can award to students who participate in the club and a blank certificate that you can print and customize to use with your own club.

Fitness Trail

Designate a trail outside on the playground or field for walking and jogging. Place a fitness exercise station or task card every 50 feet or so around the track. Students jog or walk the trail, and when they reach a fitness card, they perform the exercise shown on that card.

Pay to Play

Students jog or walk around a designated area. After completing each lap, they receive a Healthy Body Benefit Buck. When students have collected enough money, they can purchase another activity to play by paying the banker (the teacher). You can decide the cost of each activity; a good rule of thumb is to charge 5 dollars to play for 5 minutes. The DVD includes eight Benefit Bucks to use during this activity.

Seasonal Events and Health Observances

During the school year, you can take advantage of seasonal events and special health observances, in which certain months, weeks, or days are devoted to promoting good fitness and health, sound nutrition, and physical activity. Look through the list of events and observances, and choose one to spotlight during each Wellness Week. The DVD includes signs to promote the events and observances.

Step 8: Assessment

How will you know if the Wellness Week was successful? An approved school wellness policy requires assessment. Appendix B provides seven tools that help you assess the effectiveness of the Wellness Weeks that you conduct as part of the **Fitness for Life: Elementary School** program. Consider doing an assessment using these tools, or revise some of the materials and conduct an assessment that meets your school's needs. These tools are also available on the DVD in the following folder.

 General → Assessments

Classroom Teacher Program Assessment Tool

Physical Education Teacher Program Assessment Tool

Student Video Activity Ratings

Wellness Coordinator Program Assessment Tool

Family Wellness Week Assessment

Family Physical Activity and Nutrition Questionnaire

Analysis Form for Assessments

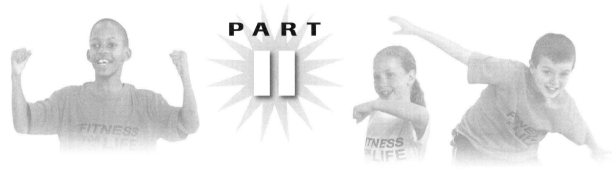

PART

II

WELLNESS WEEK PLANS

● ● ● ● ● ● ● ● ● ● ● ● ● ● ● ● ● ● ●

Part II outlines specific steps that the wellness coordinator should follow when planning and conducting Wellness Week 1 (page 27), Wellness Week 2 (page 37), Wellness Week 3 (page 45), and Wellness Week 4 (page 53).

Before reading this section, be sure to read part I (especially "Implementing the Program," starting on page 15) and familiarize yourself with the videos and resources on the DVD that accompanies this guide.

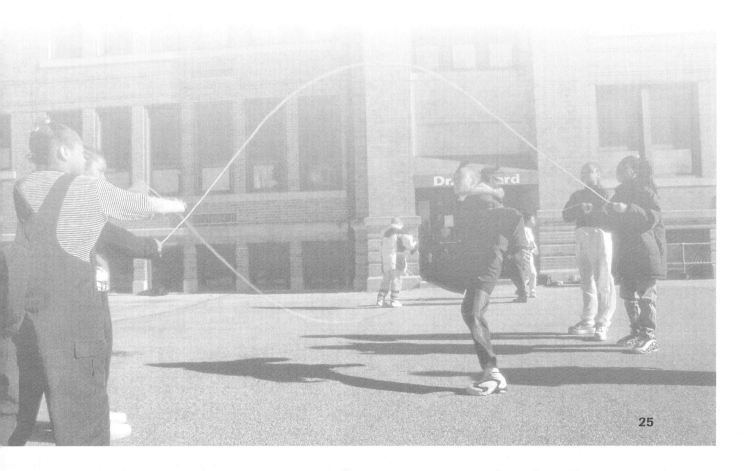

PLANNING FOR WELLNESS WEEK

1

Fitness for Life
Elementary School

This section of the guide includes all of the information that you, the wellness coordinator, will need for Wellness Week 1. It provides the themes for the week along with step by step directions for organizing activities and conducting programs. You can print a checklist from the DVD (found in the following folder) that summarizes the steps to help you plan and conduct the week's activities.

 General → Planning

Themes

- Physical activity theme: moderate physical activity
- Nutrition theme for K-2: fruits and vegetables (fitness foods)
- Nutrition theme for 3-5: fruits and vegetables (eat 5 a day)
- Nutrition theme for 6: fruits and vegetables (you are what you eat)

Step 1: Prepare Staff

One week before Wellness Week 1, you should do the following:

- Remind the physical education teacher, if there is one, to teach Warm-Up Lesson Plan 1, using the lesson plan and DVD in the *Physical Education Lesson Plans* book.

- Remind the classroom teachers about the upcoming Wellness Week. Encourage them to use the classroom guides to conduct Wellness Week activity breaks and other activities. Encourage classroom teachers to decorate their rooms with Wellness Week 1 signs.

- Remind other school staff (e.g., cafeteria, office) of upcoming Wellness Week activities.

Step 2: Distribute Newsletters

Determine whether the Wellness Week newsletter will be distributed centrally by you (via print or the Web), by the classroom teachers, or by the physical education teacher. All the newsletters are provided on the DVD in this guide, on the DVDs in the classroom guides, and on the resource CD-ROM in the *Physical Education Lesson Plans* book. Thus, it is easy for anyone—you, the classroom teachers, or the physical education teacher—to distribute the proper newsletter during each Wellness Week.

If you will be distributing the newsletter, follow these steps.

- Open the Wellness Week 1 newsletter from the DVD in this guide. Follow the folder path that follows.

- Customize the newsletter using your school's name, the date, and any other information specific to your school. The newsletter file includes directions for making changes.

WEEK 1

- Choose a day during Wellness Week for distribution.
- Print the newsletters or prepare a version to be e-mailed or posted online.
- Distribute the newsletters. Give them to students to take home, send them via e-mail, or post them to the Web. If possible, use more than one form of distribution to increase the chances that you will reach everyone.

 Wellness Week 1 → Newsletter

Step 3: Post General and Weekly Signs

The messages and concepts in the general signs and the weekly signs are discussed in the classroom and in physical education class and are included in video messages. Posting signs will help reinforce these important nutrition and physical activity messages and concepts. If possible, have members of the office staff assist you. You may also want to ask students to help print and decorate the signs before posting.

General Signs

Before or after school on the Friday before Wellness Week 1, post the general signs in the suggested locations. Post as many of these signs as you wish. After Wellness Week 1 is done, save the general signs to use again for subsequent Wellness Weeks. Remember that the General Signs folder on the DVD includes a blank horizontal sign and a blank vertical sign so that you can make your own signs that feature the **Fitness for Life: Elementary School** design.

Suggested locations for posting the general signs include near the school entrance (G1 and G2), in the cafeteria (G4, G5, and G10), in the hallways (G5 and G7), in the school gym (G9), in other common areas (G1, G2, G3, G8, and G9), and in the location where the TEAM Time activity will be held (G6 and G7).

 General → General Signs

G1: Fitness for Life: Elementary School

G2: Wellness Week

G3: Physical Activity Pyramid for Kids

G4: MyPyramid for Kids

G5: Eat Well Wednesday

G6: TEAM Time: Together Everyone Achieves More

G7: Get Fit Friday

G8: Healthy mind, healthy body, healthy heart . . . let's start!

G9: ABCs of Physical Activity

G10: ABCs of Nutrition

Weekly Signs

In addition to the general signs, the DVD includes specific signs that are meant for Wellness Week 1. These signs contain messages that relate to the week's themes. The signs are saved together in one file so you can easily print them all at once. Post the weekly signs in hallways throughout the school.

 Wellness Week 1 → Weekly Signs

Physical Activity Pyramid: Moderate activity every day!

Green is for veggies, red is for fruits!

Whatever you love to play, get 60 minutes every day!

Move your muscles when you work and play!

The more you practice, the better you get!

Keep on trying. The more you try, the better you get!

Eat the rainbow way: every color, every day!

Play safely!

I can, you can, we all can work together!

Eat 5 a day, every day!

Start with safety! Finish with fun!

Fun for me, fun for all!

Step 4: Encourage Active Playgrounds

The Active Playgrounds sign file contains signs related to getting kids active while on the playground. The signs are saved together in one file so you can easily print them all at once. Consider saving them in a folder to reuse during other

GENERAL SIGNS

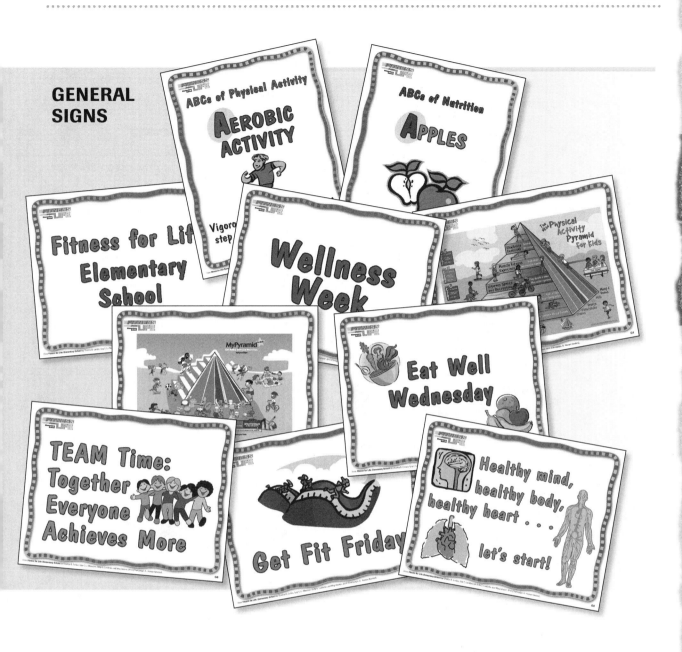

Wellness Weeks. If possible, have members of the office staff assist you. You may also want to ask students to help with printing and decorating the signs before posting.

Use the following steps to help encourage more active behavior on the playground.

- Print the active playground signs.
- Post the signs near the doors to the playground. Encourage teachers to call attention to these signs.
- Ask staff members or teachers to make some activity equipment available during recess and lunch.

- Create an activity bin that has balls, jump ropes, and so on that can be wheeled out to activity areas.
- Encourage teachers (both classroom and physical education) to help students stay active on the playground by having them do some of the physical activities that they learned during Wellness Week. Encourage activity in tether ball, Four Square, and other sports and activities typically done on your school playground.
- Ask playground supervisors to verbally encourage active play.

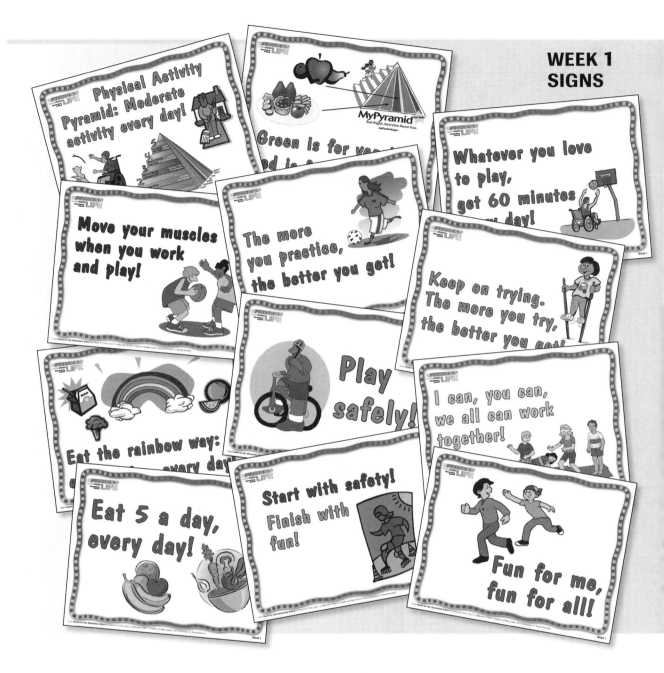

WEEK 1 SIGNS

 General → Active Playground Signs

Active play area ahead: Get moving!

You have a green light! Get your body running!

No sitting, no standing! Get active, get moving!

Choose to be active!

Start your engine and get moving now!

Caution: Children moving ahead!

Don't sit, get fit!

Get off your seat and move your feet!

Step 5: Coordinate Eat Well Wednesday Activities

Eat Well Wednesday is devoted to nutrition. Consistent with the weekly theme, the focus of the Eat Well Wednesday activity for Wellness Week 1 is on fruits and vegetables. Make contact with cafeteria workers and other staff ahead of Wellness Week 1 to allow time for the Eat Well Wednesday activity. In addition, print and post the cafeteria signs as desired, and save them for use in subsequent Wellness Weeks.

ACTIVE PLAYGROUND SIGNS

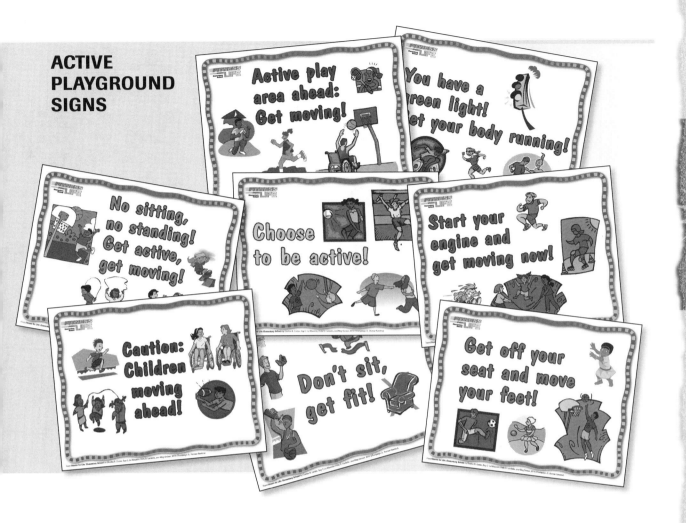

A to Z Fruit and Vegetable Bar

This activity will expose students to a wide variety of fruits and vegetables and encourage them to choose wisely, making healthy food choices. Many kids and families do not eat or buy a variety of fruits or vegetables. A diet rich in fruits and vegetables promotes immune and circulatory system health. Messages for reinforcing the weekly nutrition theme can be found on the table tent signs on the DVD.

Preparation

- Work with staff (ahead of Wellness Week 1) to provide a fruit and vegetable bar on Eat Well Wednesday.
- Work with staff to make placards for each of the fruits and vegetables that are available on the food bar so the children can identify what they are eating. If you have ESL students, provide translations in other languages.

- Print the week 1 tent signs from the DVD. They are saved together in one file.

 Wellness Week 1→ Tent Signs

Eat the rainbow way: every color, every day!

Fruits and vegetables: Eat 5 to 9 a day!

Suggestions

Extend the activity to last all week by focusing on five or six different fruits and vegetables each day. For example, Monday might feature fruits and vegetables that begin with the letters A to E (such as apples, bananas, corn, dates, and eggplant), Tuesday can feature those beginning with F to K, and so on.

Eat Well Wednesday classroom activities can also be planned. The classroom guides provide outlines for discussions that promote the Wellness Week 1 nutrition theme.

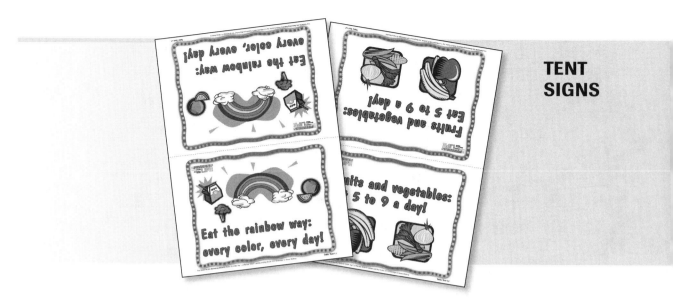

TENT SIGNS

Cafeteria Signs

The DVD includes general cafeteria signs related to nutrition. The messages and concepts in the signs are discussed in the classroom and in physical education class and are included in video messages. Posting signs will help reinforce these important nutrition and physical activity messages and concepts.

Review the signs, which are saved together in one file in the Cafeteria Signs folder on the DVD, and post as many as desired in the cafeteria during Wellness Week. You can also have students decorate the signs before posting. Consider printing all the cafeteria signs at once and saving them for use in subsequent Wellness Weeks.

In addition, the General Signs folder contains a file called G10: ABCs of Nutrition, which is a set of 26 signs (one for each letter of the alphabet) that feature nutrition images and messages. During any Wellness Week, you can use the ABCs of Nutrition signs along with, or instead of, the cafeteria signs.

 General → General Signs

　G10: ABCs of Nutrition

 General → Cafeteria Signs

　Orange is for grains!

Green is for veggies!

Red is for fruits!

Blue is for milk products!

Purple is for meat and beans!

Yellow is for oils. Use them wisely!

Life is full of choices. Choose healthy foods!

Be wise. Eat well and exercise!

Food is fuel for learning and moving. Choose wisely!

Did you eat the rainbow way today?

Eat the rainbow way: every color, every day!

Did you eat your 5 to 9 today?

Make half your grains whole!

Protein power! Get strong, live long!

You are what you eat. Choose wisely!

Avoid empty calories!

Step 6: Coordinate Get Fit Friday Activities

For Wellness Week 1, the Get Fit Friday activity is TEAM Time 1: School Walk. This activity emphasizes the weekly physical activity theme (moderate physical activity) and the concept of TEAM: Together Everyone Achieves More.

CAFETERIA SIGNS

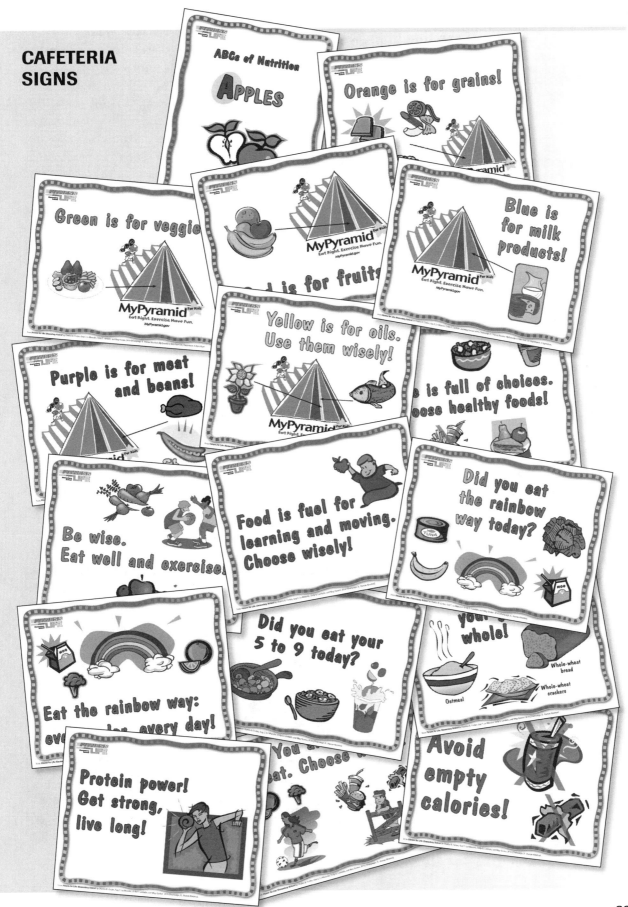

ABCs of Nutrition
APPLES

Orange is for grains!

Green is for veggies

MyPyramid For Kids
Eat Right. Exercise Have Fun.
MyPyramid.gov

Blue is for milk products!

MyPyramid For Kids
Eat Right. Exercise Have Fun.
MyPyramid.gov

MyPyramid For Kids
Eat Right. Exercise Have Fun.
MyPyramid.gov

d is for fruits

Purple is for meat and beans!

Yellow is for oils. Use them wisely!

MyPyramid For Kids
Eart Right. E

e is full of choices.
oose healthy foods!

Be wise.
Eat well and exercise

Food is fuel for learning and moving.
Choose wisely!

Did you eat the rainbow way today?

TUNA

MOO

Eat the rainbow way:
ev   every day!

Did you eat your 5 to 9 today?

whole!

Whole-wheat bread

Oatmeal

Whole-wheat crackers

Protein power!
Get strong, live long!

LIFE

You a
eat. Choose

Avoid empty calories!

33

TEAM Time 1: School Walk

When school begins, all students meet to do a 10-minute school walk. The goal is to have all students work together to get some of their 60 minutes of daily activity as recommended by national standards. The physical activity theme of Wellness Week 1 is moderate physical activity, and walking is a good moderate activity. Evidence suggests that activity at the beginning of the school day can enhance learning in the classroom (Hillman et al., 2009a; Hillman et al., 2009b; Le Masurier & Corbin, 2006; Ratey, 2008; Smith & Lounsbery, 2009).

TEAM Time 1: School Walk uses two tracks on the DVD: an instructional video that shows how one wellness coordinator conducts the activity and a music track that you can play when you lead your school in the activity. In addition, TEAM Time 1 uses a file of printable resources (a sample outline to follow and an arrow sign) that are saved together in one file in the following folder.

 Wellness Week 1 → TEAM Time

Messages

- Moderate physical activity
- TEAM: Together Everyone Achieves More

Preparation

Follow these steps to prepare for TEAM Time 1: School Walk:

- Familiarize yourself with the activity. Watch the instructional video on the DVD, which shows how one wellness coordinator conducts a School Walk.

- Print copies of the arrow sign from the DVD. Post the signs in the hallways of the school or outside. The arrows should clearly label the path of the walk.

- Show at least one teacher the path of the school walk. That teacher will lead the students and other teachers when the walk begins.

- Preview the School Walk music track on the DVD so that you are familiar with it. You may also use track 13 of the music CD in *Physical Education Lesson Plans*. However, because track 13 lasts only 5 minutes, you will have to play it twice for the 10-minute walk.

- On the day of the walk, arrange to have a DVD or CD player to play the music for the walk. You may wish to place a microphone near the DVD or CD speakers to allow the sound to be played on the school's sound system. You may also arrange other music and a method of playing it through the school sound system or use a strategically placed boombox.

Activity

- Print a copy of the School Walk sample outline from the DVD resources, or use the one on page 35.

- After students report to class and roll is taken, teachers lead students to the gym, multipurpose room, or outside. If the gym or multipurpose room is not big enough to accommodate all students, you might want to do the activity at the beginning of the day for half the students and again after lunch for the other half.

- Have classroom teachers available to monitor their own classes and encourage

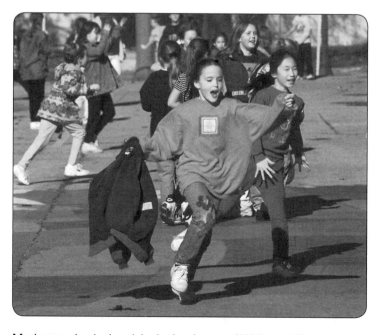

Moderate physical activity is the theme of Wellness Week 1.

active participation. Ask classroom teachers ahead of time to be ready to lead their classes in the walk when you cue them.

• Welcome students, give motivational comments, and start the event using procedures similar to those used by the wellness coordinator in the instructional video. You can use the sample outline to guide you.

• Make daily announcements or have the principal make daily announcements if there are any.

SAMPLE OUTLINE

Opening Comments

"Good morning, everybody." (Kids respond with "Good morning." Put a hand up behind your ear to indicate that they are not loud enough.) "I can't hear you. Let's try that again. Good morning, everybody!" (Kids respond with "Good morning!")

"Welcome to TEAM Time. TEAM stands for 'Together Everyone Achieves More.' Today we are going to do a School Walk with music. Each day, kids should do at least 60 minutes of physical activity. Moderate activity such as walking is good for you. A 10-minute walk today will help you get started with your 60 minutes of activity and will help you to do well in your school work when we are finished.

"When we walk, we will walk as a school team. Your teacher will set the pace. Walk at the same pace as your teacher, and stay with your class. You can talk with friends as you walk as long as you keep up.

"At the end of the walk, we will come back here before going back to your classrooms.

"When the music begins, we will get started. When I say the name of your teacher, he or she will begin walking. Follow your teacher. The arrow signs on the walls will help you know where to walk."

Activity

Start the music and begin calling out teachers' names. Teachers walk through the halls with their classes, following the path marked by the arrow signs. Continue until all classes are walking.

Closing Comments

After 10 minutes, stop the music and say, "Keep walking. When you reach the starting point, wait with your teacher until all children are finished."

After all students have returned, say, "Great job! You worked well as a team when doing this TEAM Time activity."

"OK, let's keep working as a team. It's time to go back to your classrooms, and remember that Together Everyone Achieves More. Kindergarten students, follow your teacher back to your classroom." (Allow time.) "Now the first-grade students." (Allow time.) "Now the second-grade students." (Allow time. Continue in this manner until all grades are dismissed. Alternatively, you may use a list of teachers' names to let classes know when to begin walking back to their classrooms.)

WEEK 1

WEEK 1

- Use a list of teachers' names to call out the order in which classes will begin the School Walk. Call the name of the teacher who previously learned the correct path so that he or she can lead the School Walk through the halls.

- Play the School Walk music track on the DVD.

- After everyone has returned to the starting point, congratulate the students. Then dismiss students by calling the names of their teachers, who leave with the students as their names are called.

Step 7: Coordinate Special Celebrations

Appendix A of this guide contains complete descriptions of several Wellness Week celebration activities. Encourage teachers and parents to conduct one or more of these celebrations, or if time allows, coordinate the event of your choice. Events from which you may choose include the following:

- Brain Walk
- Family Fun Night
- Fitness-a-Thon

- Fun Run/Walk (could be tied to Halloween or Thanksgiving)
- GYM (Get Yourself Moving) Club
- Fitness Trail
- Pay to Play
- Seasonal events and health observances

Step 8: Assess Responses

Use one or more of the assessment tools to assess student, teacher, and parent responses to the Wellness Week and other school wellness activities. The assessment tools can be found on the DVD or in appendix B (page 92).

 General → Assessments

Classroom Teacher Program Assessment Tool

Physical Education Teacher Program Assessment Tool

Student Video Activity Ratings

Wellness Coordinator Program Assessment Tool

Family Wellness Week Assessment

Family Physical Activity and Nutrition Questionnaire

Analysis Form for Assessments

PLANNING FOR WELLNESS WEEK

2

Fitness for Life Elementary School

This section of the guide includes all of the information that you will need for Wellness Week 2. It provides the themes for the week along with step by step directions for organizing activities and conducting programs. You can print a checklist from the DVD (found in the following folder) that summarizes the steps to help you plan and conduct the week's activities.

 General → Planning

Themes

- Physical activity theme: vigorous physical activity (vigorous aerobics, sports, and recreation)
- Nutrition theme for K-2: grains and foods with fat
- Nutrition theme for 3-5: grains and empty calories
- Nutrition theme for 6: grains and high-calorie foods

Step 1: Prepare Staff

One week before Wellness Week 2, you should do the following:

- Remind the physical education teacher, if there is one, to teach Warm-Up Lesson Plan 2, using the lesson plan and DVD in the *Physical Education Lesson Plans* book.
- Remind the classroom teachers about the upcoming Wellness Week. Encourage them

to use the classroom guides to conduct Wellness Week activity breaks and other activities. Encourage classroom teachers to decorate their rooms with Wellness Week 2 signs.

- Remind other school staff (e.g., cafeteria, office) of upcoming Wellness Week activities.

Step 2: Distribute Newsletters

Determine whether the Wellness Week newsletter will be distributed centrally by you (via print or the Web), by the classroom teachers, or by the physical education teacher. All the newsletters are provided on the DVD in this guide, on the DVDs in the classroom guides, and on the resource CD-ROM in the *Physical Education Lesson Plans* book. Thus, it is easy for anyone—you, the classroom teachers, or the physical education teacher—to distribute the proper newsletter during each Wellness Week.

If you will be distributing the newsletter, follow these steps.

- Open the Wellness Week 2 newsletter from the DVD in this guide. Follow the folder path that follows.
- Customize the newsletter using your school's name, the date, and any other information specific to your school. The

newsletter file includes directions for making changes.

- Choose a day during Wellness Week for distribution.
- Print the newsletters or prepare a version to be e-mailed or posted online.
- Distribute the newsletters. Give them to students to take home, send them via e-mail, or post them to the Web. If possible, use more than one form of distribution to increase the chances that you will reach everyone.

 Wellness Week 2 → Newsletter

Step 3: Post General and Weekly Signs

The messages and concepts in the general signs and the weekly signs are discussed in the classroom and in physical education class and are included in video messages. Posting signs will help reinforce these important nutrition and physical activity messages and concepts. If possible, have members of the office staff assist you. You may also want to ask students to help print and decorate the signs before posting.

General Signs

Before or after school on the Friday before Wellness Week 2, post the general signs in the suggested locations. Post as many of these signs as you wish. After Wellness Week 2 is done, save the general signs to use again for subsequent Wellness Weeks. Remember that the General Signs folder on the DVD includes a blank horizontal sign and a blank vertical sign so that you can make your own signs that feature the **Fitness for Life: Elementary School** design.

The general signs are listed below. You can see thumbnails of the general signs on page 29.

Suggested locations for posting the general signs include near the school entrance (G1 and G2), in the cafeteria (G4, G5, and G10), in the hallways (G5 and G7), in the school gym (G9), in other common areas (G1, G2, G3, G8, and G9), and in the location where the TEAM Time activity will be held (G6 and G7).

 General → General Signs

G1: Fitness for Life: Elementary School
G2: Wellness Week
G3: Physical Activity Pyramid for Kids
G4: MyPyramid for Kids
G5: Eat Well Wednesday
G6: TEAM Time: Together Everyone Achieves More
G7: Get Fit Friday
G8: Healthy mind, healthy body, healthy heart . . . let's start!
G9: ABCs of Physical Activity
G10: ABCs of Nutrition

Weekly Signs

In addition to the general signs, the DVD includes specific signs that are meant for Wellness Week 2. These signs contain messages that relate to the week's themes. The signs are saved together in one file so you can easily print them all at once. Post the weekly signs in hallways throughout the school.

 Wellness Week 2 → Weekly Signs

Physical Activity Pyramid: Make some activity vigorous!

Orange is for grains!

Avoid empty calories!

A healthy body needs a healthy mind!

Get your body moving!

The more you practice, the better you play; practice, practice every day!

Making your heart beat fast helps your body last!

A healthy heart is a happy heart!

Exercising your heart daily really pays. Your heart will thank you in many ways!

Keep on going to get fit. Never give up! Never quit!

Play for a good day!

Activity + academics = a winning combination!

Build skills, have fun!

Make half your grains whole!

Get some aerobic activity every day!

Show respect—follow the golden rule!

To be fit, you must think FITT!

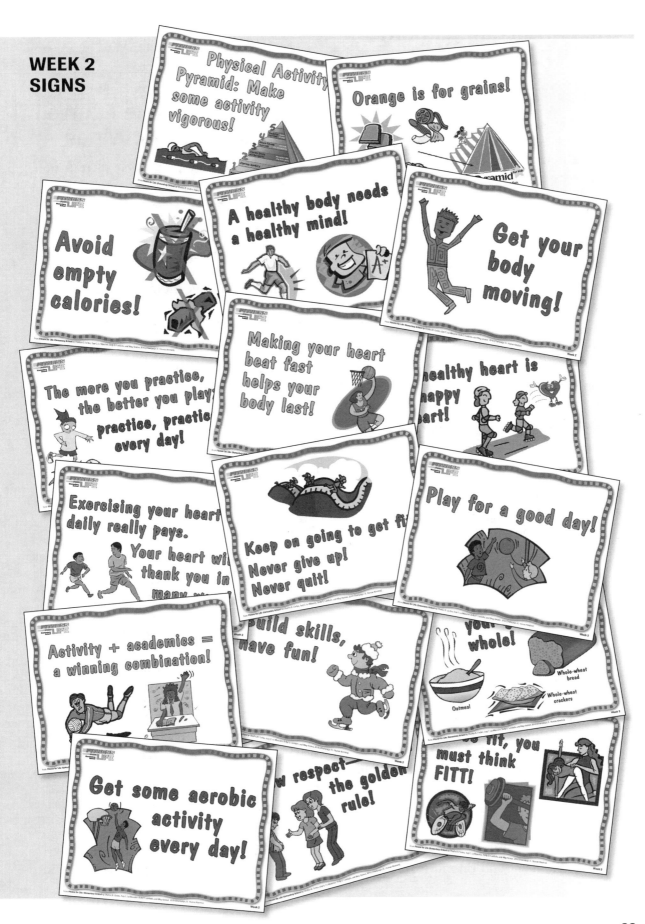

WEEK 2

Step 4: Encourage Active Playgrounds

The Active Playgrounds sign file contains signs related to getting kids active while on the playground. The signs are saved together in one file so you can easily print them all at once. Consider saving them in a folder to reuse during other Wellness Weeks. If possible, have members of the office staff assist you. You may also want to ask students to help with printing and decorating the signs before posting.

Use the following steps to help encourage more active behavior on the playground.

- Print the active playground signs.
- Post the signs near the doors to the playground. Encourage teachers to call attention to these signs.
- Ask staff members or teachers to make some activity equipment available during recess and lunch.
- Create an activity bin that has balls, jump ropes, and so on that can be wheeled out to activity areas.
- Encourage teachers (both classroom and physical education) to help students stay active on the playground by having them do some of the physical activities that they learned during Wellness Week. Encourage activity in tether ball, Four Square, and other sports and activities typically done on your school playground.
- Ask playground supervisors to verbally encourage active play.

The Active Playground signs are listed below. You can see thumbnails of the signs on page 31.

 General → Active Playground Signs

Active play area ahead: Get moving!

You have a green light! Get your body running!

No sitting, no standing! Get active, get moving!

Choose to be active!

Start your engine and get moving now!

Caution: Children moving ahead!

Don't sit, get fit!

Get off your seat and move your feet!

Step 5: Coordinate Eat Well Wednesday Activities

Eat Well Wednesday is devoted to nutrition. Consistent with the weekly theme, the focus of the Eat Well Wednesday activity for Wellness Week 2 is on a healthy breakfast, with an emphasis on grains along with other foods. Make contact with cafeteria workers and other staff ahead of Wellness Week 2 to allow time for the following Eat Well Wednesday activity.

Promoting a Healthy Breakfast Program

On Eat Well Wednesday, promote a healthy breakfast by offering only healthy breakfast choices. Examples include a bowl of whole-wheat cereal with fruit and low-fat white milk, or scrambled eggs and a whole-wheat English muffin. Help students have healthy choices that let them make half their grains whole. Messages for reinforcing the weekly nutrition theme can be found on the table tent signs on the DVD.

Preparation

- Work with staff (ahead of Wellness Week 2) to plan the Healthy Breakfast activity.
- Print the week 2 tent signs from the DVD. They are saved together in one file.

 Wellness Week 2 → Tent Signs

Eat breakfast: Make healthy choices!

Make half your grains whole!

Suggestions

Eat Well Wednesday classroom activities can also be planned. The classroom guides provide outlines for discussions that promote the Wellness Week 2 nutrition theme.

Cafeteria Signs

The DVD includes general cafeteria signs related to nutrition. The messages and concepts

TENT SIGNS

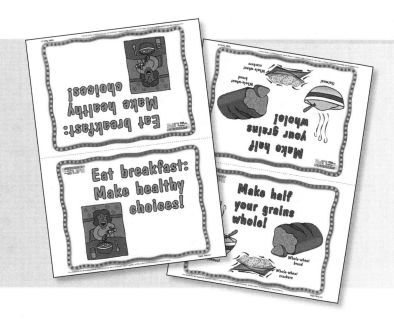

in the signs are discussed in the classroom and in physical education class and are included in video messages. Posting signs will help reinforce these important nutrition and physical activity messages and concepts.

Review the signs, which are saved together in one file in the Cafeteria Signs folder on the DVD, and post as many as desired in the cafeteria during Wellness Week. You can also have students decorate the signs before posting. Consider printing all the cafeteria signs at once and saving them for use in subsequent Wellness Weeks.

In addition, the General Signs folder contains a file called G10: ABCs of Nutrition, which is a set of 26 signs (one for each letter of the alphabet) that feature nutrition images and messages. During any Wellness Week, you can use the ABCs of Nutrition signs along with, or instead of, the cafeteria signs.

You can see thumbnails of the cafeteria signs on page 33.

 General → General Signs

   G10: ABCs of Nutrition

 General → Cafeteria Signs

   Orange is for grains!
   Green is for veggies!

Red is for fruits!

Blue is for milk products!

Purple is for meat and beans!

Yellow is for oils. Use them wisely!

Life is full of choices. Choose healthy foods!

Be wise. Eat well and exercise!

Food is fuel for learning and moving. Choose wisely!

Did you eat the rainbow way today?

Eat the rainbow way: every color, every day!

Did you eat your 5 to 9 today?

Make half your grains whole!

Protein power! Get strong, live long!

You are what you eat. Choose wisely!

Avoid empty calories!

Step 6: Coordinate Get Fit Friday Activities

For Wellness Week 2, the Get Fit Friday activity is TEAM Time 2: Big Kids Lead. This activity emphasizes the weekly physical activity theme: vigorous physical activity (vigorous aerobics, sports, and recreation) and the concept of TEAM: Together Everyone Achieves More.

WEEK 2

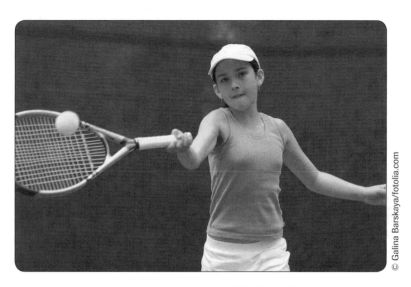

© Galina Barskaya/fotolia.com

Vigorous physical activity is the theme of Wellness Week 2.

TEAM Time 2: Big Kids Lead

During the first 10 minutes of school, all students will perform an activity led by the wellness coordinator and specially selected fifth- and sixth-grade students. The goal is to have all students work together to get some of their 60 minutes of daily activity as recommended by national standards. The theme of the second Wellness Week is vigorous physical activity (vigorous aerobics, sports, and recreation) so some of this activity is vigorous activity. Evidence suggests that activity at the beginning of the school day can enhance learning in the classroom (Hillman et al., 2009a; Hillman et al., 2009b; Le Masurier & Corbin, 2006; Ratey, 2008; Smith & Lounsbery, 2009).

TEAM Time 2: Big Kids Lead uses four tracks on the DVD: an instructional video that shows how one wellness coordinator conducts the activity and three routines (a warm-up, an activity called Colors, and a cool-down) that you can play when you lead your school. In addition, TEAM Time 2 uses a file of printable resources (a sample outline to follow and the specific exercises in each routine) that are saved together in one file in the following folder.

 Wellness Week 2 → TEAM Time

Messages

- Vigorous physical activity (vigorous aerobics, sports, and recreation)

- TEAM (Together Everyone Achieves More)

Preparation

To prepare for TEAM Time 2: Big Kids Lead, the following steps are recommended.

- Familiarize yourself with the activity. Watch the instructional video on the DVD, which shows how one wellness coordinator conducts the activity.
- Familiarize yourself with the resources.
- Select some fifth- and sixth-grade students to help you lead the activity.
- Plan a practice session with the student leaders before the actual event. Use the warm-up, Colors, and cool-down videos on the DVD to learn the movements for each part of the activity. Help the student leaders learn the movements so that they can help you lead on the day of the event. You may also want to have the students learn the words to the Colors song.
- You may also want to distribute the words to the classroom teachers beforehand so that students can sing along.
- You may want to have the music teacher help the student leaders learn the words to the Colors routine.
- Arrange for a DVD player on the day of the event. If you have a computer and computer projector, you can use them to project a large image.

Activity

- Print a copy of the TEAM Time 2 sample outline from the DVD, or use the one on the next page.
- Set up a DVD player (or computer and computer projector) in the location where TEAM Time will be held.
- If possible, place a microphone by the DVD speaker so that music for TEAM Time is loud enough for all to hear. Turn the DVD volume up loud.

WEEK 2

- You may want to turn the screen of the DVD away from the students so that they focus on watching you and the student leaders rather than everyone watching the routine on the screen.

- Have classroom teachers available to monitor their own classes and encourage active participation.

- After students report to class and roll is taken, teachers lead students to the gym, the multipurpose room, or outside. If the gym or multipurpose room is not big enough to accommodate all the students, you might want to do the activity at the beginning of the day for half the students and again after lunch for the other half.

- Welcome students, give motivational comments, and start the event using procedures similar to those used by the wellness coordinator in the instructional video. You can use the sample outline to guide you.

SAMPLE OUTLINE

Opening Comments

"Good morning, everybody." (Kids respond with "Good morning." Put a hand up behind your ear to indicate that they are not loud enough.) "I can't hear you. Let's try that again. Good morning, everybody!" (Kids respond with "Good morning!")

"Welcome to TEAM Time. TEAM stands for 'Together Everyone Achieves More.' We are going to do some fun activities as a team to get us ready for the school day. At the end of the routine, we are going to do a chant. Let's practice it so that you are ready when the time comes.

"I'll say it first and then you say it: Stay active, eat well." (Kids respond with "Stay active, eat well.") "Say it again: Stay active, eat well." (Kids respond with "Stay active, eat well.")

"Now we're going to do the activity. Just watch what we do and follow along. Don't worry if you make a mistake. Just do the best that you can. You can sing or hum along with the music if you like."

Activity

Conduct Big Kids Lead with the warm-up, Colors, and cool-down videos. During the activity, periodically repeat the following statements to encourage students: "Good job. Nice work. Keep trying, you are getting it. Way to go. Stick with it."

Closing Comments

Have students repeat the chant at the end of the routine: "Stay active, eat well."

After the routine, consider using these comments: "Great job! You worked well as a team when doing the TEAM Time activity.

"OK, let's keep working as a team. It's time to go back to your classrooms, and remember that Together Everyone Achieves More. Kindergarten students, follow your teacher back to your classroom." (Allow time.) "Now the first-grade students." (Allow time.) "Now the second-grade students." (Allow time. Continue in this manner until all grades are dismissed. Alternatively, you may use a list of teachers' names to let classes know when to begin walking back to their classrooms.)

WEEK 2

- Make daily announcements or have the principal make daily announcements if there are any.
- Lead the TEAM Time 2 routine with the help of the fifth- and sixth-grade leaders. Place these leaders around the TEAM Time area so that they are visible to as many children as possible. Encourage students to watch you or your student leaders. If they cannot easily see a leader, encourage them to follow other students who can see a leader.
- Play the warm-up, Colors, and cool-down videos on the DVD to cue your movements and the movements of student leaders.
- When the routine is finished, congratulate the students. Then dismiss students by calling the names of teachers, who leave with their students as their names are called.

Step 7: Coordinate Special Celebrations

Appendix A of this guide contains complete descriptions of several Wellness Week celebration activities. Encourage teachers and parents to conduct one or more of these celebrations, or if time allows, coordinate the event of your choice. Events from which you may choose include the following:

- Brain Walk
- Family Fun Night
- Fitness-a-Thon
- Fun Run/Walk (could be tied to Halloween or Thanksgiving)
- GYM (Get Yourself Moving) Club
- Fitness Trail
- Pay to Play
- Seasonal events and health observances

Step 8: Assess Responses

Use one or more of the assessment tools to assess student, teacher, and parent responses to the Wellness Week and other school wellness activities. The assessment tools can be found on the DVD or in appendix B (page 92).

 General → Assessments

Classroom Teacher Program Assessment Tool

Physical Education Teacher Program Assessment Tool

Student Video Activity Ratings

Wellness Coordinator Program Assessment Tool

Family Wellness Week Assessment

Family Physical Activity and Nutrition Questionnaire

Analysis Form for Assessments

PLANNING FOR WELLNESS WEEK 3

Fitness for Life Elementary School

This section of the guide includes all of the information that you will need for Wellness Week 3. It provides the themes for the week along with step by step directions for organizing activities and conducting programs. You can print a checklist from the DVD (found in the following folder) that summarizes the steps to help you plan and conduct the week's activities.

 General → Planning

Themes

- Physical activity theme: muscle fitness and flexibility exercises
- Nutrition theme for K-2: foods for strong bones and muscles
- Nutrition theme for 3-5: protein power
- Nutrition theme for 6: protein is important

Step 1: Prepare Staff

One week before Wellness Week 3, you should do the following:

- Remind the physical education teacher, if there is one, to teach Warm-Up Lesson Plan 3, using the lesson plan and DVD in the *Physical Education Lesson Plans* book.
- Remind the classroom teachers about the upcoming Wellness Week. Encourage them to use the classroom guides to conduct Wellness Week activity breaks and other activities. Encourage classroom teachers

to decorate their rooms with Wellness Week 3 signs.
- Remind other school staff (e.g., cafeteria, office) of upcoming Wellness Week activities.

Step 2: Distribute Newsletters

Determine whether the Wellness Week newsletter will be distributed centrally by you (via print or the Web), by the classroom teachers, or by the physical education teacher. All the newsletters are provided on the DVD in this guide, on the DVDs in the classroom guides, and on the resource CD-ROM in the *Physical Education Lesson Plans* book. Thus, it is easy for anyone—you, the classroom teachers, or the physical education teacher—to distribute the proper newsletter during each Wellness Week.

If you will be distributing the newsletter, follow these steps.

- Open the Wellness Week 3 newsletter from the DVD in this guide. Follow the folder path that follows.
- Customize the newsletter using your school's name, the date, and any other information specific to your school. The newsletter file includes directions for making changes.
- Choose a day during Wellness Week for distribution.
- Print the newsletters or prepare a version to be e-mailed or posted online.

- Distribute the newsletters. Give them to students to take home, send them via e-mail, or post them to the Web. If possible, use more than one form of distribution to increase the chances that you will reach everyone.

 Wellness Week 3 → Newsletter

Step 3: Post General and Weekly Signs

The messages and concepts in the general signs and the weekly signs are discussed in the classroom and in physical education class and are included in video messages. Posting signs will help reinforce these important nutrition and physical activity messages and concepts. If possible, have members of the office staff assist you. You may also want to ask students to help print and decorate the signs before posting.

General Signs

Before or after school on the Friday before Wellness Week 3, post the general signs in the suggested locations. Post as many of these signs as you wish. After Wellness Week 3 is done, save the general signs to use again for subsequent Wellness Weeks. Remember that the General Signs folder on the DVD includes a blank horizontal sign and a blank vertical sign so that you can make your own signs that feature the **Fitness for Life: Elementary School** design.

The general signs are listed below. You can see thumbnails of the general signs on page 29.

Suggested locations for posting the general signs include near the school entrance (G1 and G2), in the cafeteria (G4, G5, and G10), in the hallways (G5 and G7), in the school gym (G9), in other common areas (G1, G2, G3, G8, and G9), and in the location where the TEAM Time activity will be held (G6 and G7).

 General → General Signs

G1: Fitness for Life: Elementary School

G2: Wellness Week

G3: Physical Activity Pyramid for Kids

G4: MyPyramid for Kids

G5: Eat Well Wednesday

G6: TEAM Time: Together Everyone Achieves More

G7: Get Fit Friday

G8: Healthy mind, healthy body, healthy heart . . . let's start!

G9: ABCs of Physical Activity

G10: ABCs of Nutrition

Weekly Signs

In addition to the general signs, the DVD includes specific signs that are meant for Wellness Week 3. These signs contain messages that relate to the week's themes. The signs are saved together in one file so you can easily print them all at once. Post the weekly signs in hallways throughout the school.

 Wellness Week 3 → Weekly Signs

Physical Activity Pyramid: Do exercise for muscle fitness and flexibility!

Blue is for milk; purple is for meat and beans!

A healthy mind needs a healthy body!

Before you play or perform, you need to get your muscles warm!

Music helps you move!

Protein power! Get strong, live long!

We have only one body. Let's make it fit!

If it is to be, it's up to me!

Building muscle requires skill and technique; strengthen your muscles three times per week!

Protein builds cells in muscles and brains; eat your protein foods and make big gains!

Be specific; look terrific!

Don't be a character; show your character!

Follow the rules and share the ball; demonstrate fairness, respect, and teamwork to all!

There is no "I" in "team"!

Step 4: Encourage Active Playgrounds

The Active Playgrounds sign file contains signs related to getting kids active while on the playground. The signs are saved together in one file

WEEK 3 SIGNS

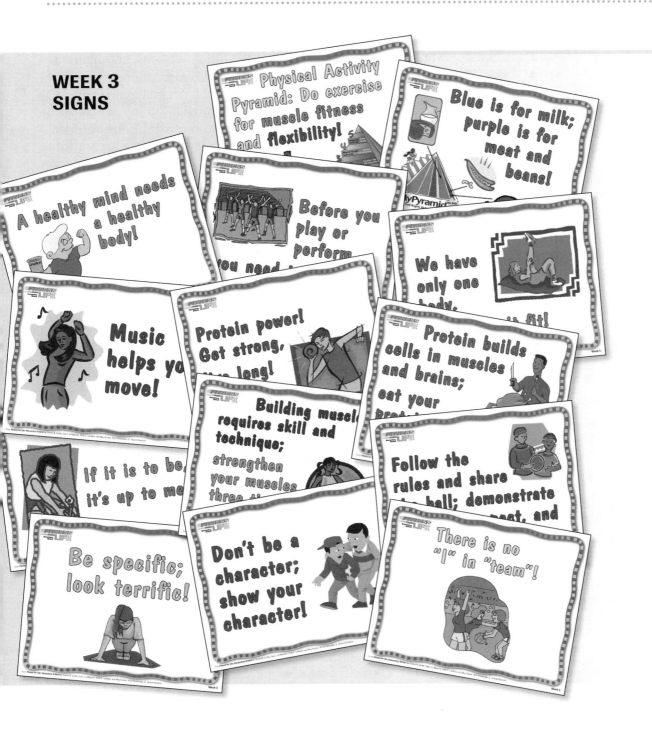

so you can easily print them all at once. Consider saving them in a folder to reuse during other Wellness Weeks. If possible, have members of the office staff assist you. You may also want to ask students to help with printing and decorating the signs before posting.

Use the following steps to help encourage more active behavior on the playground.

- Print the active playground signs.

- Post the signs near the doors to the playground. Encourage teachers to call attention to these signs.

- Ask staff members or teachers to make some activity equipment available during recess and lunch.

- Create an activity bin that has balls, jump ropes, and so on that can be wheeled out to activity areas.
- Encourage teachers (both classroom and physical education) to help students stay active on the playground by having them do some of the physical activities that they learned during Wellness Week. Encourage activity in tether ball, Four Square, and other sports and activities typically done on your school playground.
- Ask playground supervisors to verbally encourage active play.

The Active Playground signs are listed below. You can see thumbnails of the signs on page 31.

 General → Active Playground Signs

Active play area ahead: Get moving!

You have a green light! Get your body running!

No sitting, no standing! Get active, get moving!

Choose to be active!

Start your engine and get moving now!

Caution: Children moving ahead!

Don't sit, get fit!

Get off your seat and move your feet!

Step 5: Coordinate Eat Well Wednesday Activities

Eat Well Wednesday is devoted to nutrition. Consistent with the weekly theme, the focus of the Eat Well Wednesday activity for Wellness Week 3 is on protein. Make contact with cafeteria workers and other staff ahead of Wellness Week 3 to allow time for the following Eat Well Wednesday activity.

Fuel Up: Yogurt Bar

This activity promotes "protein power" by giving students an opportunity to try different types of yogurt. One serving of yogurt can provide 10 to 20 percent of daily protein needs. Depending on your school's nut policy, you might consider stirring ground walnuts, almonds, or other nuts into the yogurt to provide even more protein and make students aware of foods containing protein. Although fruit is not high in protein, it can add flavor to yogurt and promote fruit consumption. Provide a variety of fruits, including berries and peaches, to mix into the yogurt. Messages for reinforcing the weekly nutrition theme can be found on the table tent signs on the DVD.

Preparation

- Work with staff (ahead of Wellness Week 3) to plan the fruit and yogurt bar.
- Print the week 3 tent signs from the DVD. They are saved together in one file.

 Wellness Week 3 → Tent Signs

Protein power! Get strong, live long!

Foods for strong bones and muscles

Suggestions

Eat Well Wednesday classroom activities can also be planned. The classroom guides provide outlines for discussions that promote the Wellness Week 3 nutrition theme.

Cafeteria Signs

The DVD includes general cafeteria signs related to nutrition. The messages and concepts in the signs are discussed in the classroom and in physical education class and are included in video messages. Posting signs will help reinforce these important nutrition and physical activity messages and concepts.

Review the signs, which are saved together in one file in the Cafeteria Signs folder on the DVD, and post as many as desired in the cafeteria during Wellness Week. You can also have students decorate the signs before posting. Consider printing all the cafeteria signs at once and saving them for use in subsequent Wellness Weeks.

In addition, the General Signs folder contains a file called G10: ABCs of Nutrition, which is a set of 26 signs (one for each letter of the alphabet) that feature nutrition images and messages. During any Wellness Week, you can

TENT SIGNS

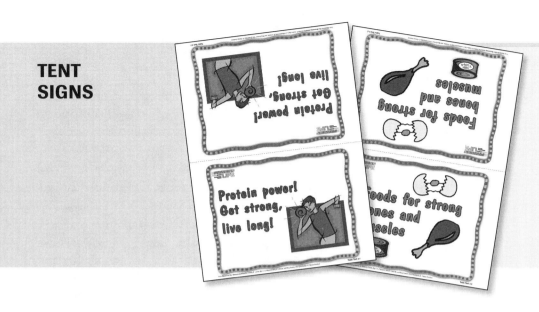

use the ABCs of Nutrition signs along with, or instead of, the cafeteria signs.

You can see thumbnails of the cafeteria signs on page 33.

 General → General Signs

G10: ABCs of Nutrition

 General → Cafeteria Signs

Orange is for grains!

Green is for veggies!

Red is for fruits!

Blue is for milk products!

Purple is for meat and beans!

Yellow is for oils. Use them wisely!

Life is full of choices. Choose healthy foods!

Be wise. Eat well and exercise!

Food is fuel for learning and moving. Choose wisely!

Did you eat the rainbow way today?

Eat the rainbow way: every color, every day!

Did you eat your 5 to 9 today?

Make half your grains whole!

Protein power! Get strong, live long!

You are what you eat. Choose wisely!

Avoid empty calories!

Step 6: Coordinate Get Fit Friday Activities

For Wellness Week 3, the Get Fit Friday activity is TEAM Time 3: Little Kids Lead. This activity emphasizes the weekly physical activity theme (muscle fitness and flexibility exercises) and the concept of TEAM: Together Everyone Achieves More.

TEAM Time 3: Little Kids Lead

During the first 10 minutes of school, all students will perform three different activities. They will be led by students from grades K-2. The goals is to have all the students work together to get some of their 60 minutes of daily activity as recommended by national standards. The theme of the third Wellness Week is muscle fitness and flexibility exercises, so some exercises of this type are included. Evidence suggests that activity at the beginning of the school day can enhance learning in the classroom (Hillman et al., 2009a; Hillman et al., 2009b; Le Masurier & Corbin, 2006; Ratey, 2008; Smith & Lounsbery, 2009).

TEAM Time 3: Little Kids Lead uses four tracks on the DVD: an instructional video that shows how one wellness coordinator conducts the activity, a routine to be performed by kindergarteners (We Get Fit), a routine to be performed by first graders (CYIM Fit), and a routine to be performed by second graders (Wave

WEEK 3

WEEK 3

It). In addition, TEAM Time 3 uses a file of printable resources (a sample outline to follow, lyrics to the three routines, and movements for the three routines) that are saved together in one file in the following folder.

 Wellness Week 3 → TEAM Time

Messages

- Muscle fitness and flexibility exercises
- TEAM (Together Everyone Achieves More)

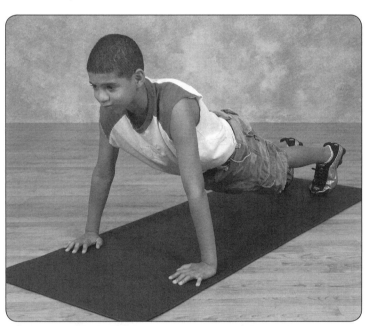

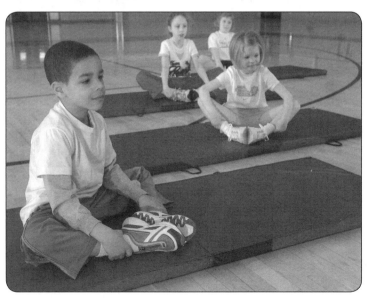

The theme of Wellness Week 3 is muscle fitness and flexibility exercises.

Preparation

To prepare for TEAM Time 3: Little Kids Lead, the following steps are recommended.

- Familiarize yourself with the activity. Watch the instructional video on the DVD, which shows how one wellness coordinator conducts this activity.
- Select some kindergarten, first-grade, and second-grade students to help you lead the TEAM Time 3 activity.
  - Check with classroom teachers to be sure that K-2 students have learned their routines for the week. Let the teachers know that their students will be performing their routine during TEAM Time.
  - You may also want to distribute the lyrics to the classroom teachers beforehand so that students can sing along.
  - If desired, plan a practice session with the student leaders before the actual event. Use the videos on the DVD to practice the movements for each routine.
  - Arrange for a DVD player on the day of the event. If you have a computer and computer projector, you can use them to project a large image.

Activity

- Print a copy of the TEAM Time 3 sample outline from the DVD, or use the one on page 52.
- Set up a DVD player (or computer and computer projector) in the location where TEAM Time will be held.
- If possible, place a microphone by the DVD speaker so that music for TEAM Time is loud enough for all to hear. Turn the DVD volume up loud.
- You may want to turn the screen of the DVD away from the students so that they focus on

watching you and the student leaders rather than everyone watching the routine on the screen.

- Have classroom teachers available to monitor their own classes and encourage active participation.

- After students report to class and roll is taken, teachers lead students to the gym, multipurpose room, or outside. If the gym or multipurpose room is not big enough to accommodate all students, you might want to do the activity at the beginning of the day for half the students and again after lunch for the other half.

- Group the kindergarten classes at the front of the TEAM Time area. Group the first graders at the back of the TEAM Time area. Group the second graders at one side of the TEAM Time area. This grouping will help you speed up the TEAM Time activity.

- Welcome students, give motivational comments, and start the event using procedures similar to those used by the wellness coordinator in the instructional video. You can use the sample outline to guide you.

- Make daily announcements or have the principal make daily announcements if there are any.

- Lead the TEAM Time 3 routine with the help of the K-2 student leaders. Encourage students to watch you or your student leaders. If they cannot easily see a leader, encourage them to follow other students who can see a leader.

- For each routine, play the corresponding video on the DVD to cue your movements and the movements of student leaders.

- When the routine is finished, congratulate the students. Then dismiss students by calling the names of teachers, who leave with their students as their names are called.

Step 7: Coordinate Special Celebrations

Appendix A of this guide contains complete descriptions of several Wellness Week celebration activities. Encourage teachers and parents to conduct one or more of these celebrations, or if time allows, coordinate the event of your choice. Events from which you may choose include the following:

- Brain Walk
- Family Fun Night
- Fitness-a-Thon
- Fun Run/Walk (could be tied to Halloween or Thanksgiving)
- GYM (Get Yourself Moving) Club
- Fitness Trail
- Pay to Play
- Seasonal events and health observances

Step 8: Assess Responses

Use one or more of the assessment tools to assess student, teacher, and parent responses to the Wellness Week and other school wellness activities. The assessment tools can be found on the DVD or in appendix B (page 92).

 General → Assessments

Classroom Teacher Program Assessment Tool

Physical Education Teacher Program Assessment Tool

Student Video Activity Ratings

Wellness Coordinator Program Assessment Tool

Family Wellness Week Assessment

Family Physical Activity and Nutrition Questionnaire

Analysis Form for Assessments

SAMPLE OUTLINE

Opening Comments

"Good morning, everybody." (Kids respond with "Good morning." Put a hand up behind your ear to indicate that they are not loud enough.) "I can't hear you. Let's try that again. Good morning, everybody!" (Kids respond with "Good morning!")

"Welcome to TEAM Time. TEAM stands for 'Together Everyone Achieves More.' We are going to do some fun activities as a team to get us ready for the school day. At the end of the routine, we are going to do a chant. Let's practice it so that you are ready when the time comes.

"I'll say it first and then you say it: Stay active, eat well." (Kids respond with "Stay active, eat well.") "Say it again: Stay active, eat well." (Kids respond with "Stay active, eat well.")

"Good job. Now let's get started. I have asked some students to help me lead. For each activity, watch what we do, and try to follow along. Don't worry if you make a mistake. Just do the best that you can."

Activity

"First the kindergarteners will lead an activity called We Get Fit." (Have all students face the kindergarten leaders.) "Help them out by doing the activity with them. It is their chance to lead. If you can't see the leaders, try to follow along with the kids in front of you." (Play We Get Fit from the DVD.)

"Now the first graders will lead an activity called CYIM Fit." (Have all students face the first-grade leaders.) "Help the first graders out by doing the activity with them. It is their chance to lead." (Play CYIM Fit from the DVD.)

"Now the second graders will lead an activity called Wave It." (Have all students face the second-grade leaders.) "Help them out by doing the activity with them. It is their chance to lead." (Play Wave It from the DVD.)

During the activities, periodically repeat the following statements to encourage students: "Good job. Nice work. Keep trying, you are getting it. Way to go. Stick with it."

Closing Comments

Have students perform the chant at the end of the routine: "Stay active, eat well."

After the routine, consider using these comments: "Great job! You worked well as a team when doing the TEAM Time activities.

"OK, let's keep working as a team. It's time to go back to your classrooms, and remember that Together Everyone Achieves More. Kindergarten students, follow your teacher back to your classroom." (Allow time.) "Now the first-grade students." (Allow time.) "Now the second-grade students." (Allow time. Continue in this manner until all grades are dismissed. Alternatively, you may use a list of teachers' names to let classes know when to begin walking back to their classrooms.)

PLANNING FOR WELLNESS WEEK

4

Fitness for Life Elementary School

This section of the guide includes all of the information that you will need for Wellness Week 4. It provides the themes for the week along with step by step directions for organizing activities and conducting programs. You can print a checklist from the DVD (found in the following folder) that summarizes the steps to help you plan and conduct the week's activities.

 General → Planning

Themes

- Physical activity theme: integration (energy balance)
- Nutrition theme for K-2: healthy foods help us move
- Nutrition theme for 3-5: balance energy in (food) with energy out (exercise)
- Nutrition theme for 6: balance calories

Step 1: Prepare Staff

One week before Wellness Week 4, you should do the following:

- Remind the physical education teacher, if there is one, to teach Warm-Up Lesson Plan 4, using the lesson plan and DVD in the *Physical Education Lesson Plans* book.
- Remind the classroom teachers about the upcoming Wellness Week. Encourage them to use the classroom guides to conduct Well-

ness Week activity breaks and other activities. Encourage classroom teachers to decorate their rooms with Wellness Week 4 signs.

- Remind other school staff (e.g., cafeteria, office) of upcoming Wellness Week activities.

Step 2: Distribute Newsletters

Determine whether the Wellness Week newsletter will be distributed centrally by you (via print or the Web), by the classroom teachers, or by the physical education teacher. All the newsletters are provided on the DVD in this guide, on the DVDs in the classroom guides, and on the resource CD-ROM in the *Physical Education Lesson Plans* book. Thus, it is easy for anyone—you, the classroom teachers, or the physical education teacher—to distribute the proper newsletter during each Wellness Week.

If you will be distributing the newsletter, follow these steps.

- Open the Wellness Week 4 newsletter from the DVD in this guide. Follow the folder path that follows.
- Customize the newsletter using your school's name, the date, and any other information specific to your school. The newsletter file includes directions for making changes.
- Choose a day during Wellness Week for distribution.

- Print the newsletters or prepare a version to be e-mailed or posted online.
- Distribute the newsletters. Give them to students to take home, send them via e-mail, or post them to the Web. If possible, use more than one form of distribution to increase the chances that you will reach everyone.

 Wellness Week 4 → Newsletter

Step 3: Post General and Weekly Signs

The messages and concepts in the general signs and the weekly signs are discussed in the classroom and in physical education class and are included in video messages. Posting signs will help reinforce these important nutrition and physical activity messages and concepts. If possible, have members of the office staff assist you. You may also want to ask students to help print and decorate the signs before posting.

General Signs

Before or after school on the Friday before Wellness Week 4, post the general signs in the suggested locations. Post as many of these signs as you wish. After Wellness Week 4 is done, save the general signs to use again for next year. Remember that the General Signs folder on the DVD includes a blank horizontal sign and a blank vertical sign so that you can make your own signs that feature the **Fitness for Life: Elementary School** design.

The general signs are listed below. You can see thumbnails of the general signs on page 29.

Suggested locations for posting the general signs include near the school entrance (G1 and G2), in the cafeteria (G4, G5, and G10), in the hallways (G5 and G7), in the school gym (G9), in other common areas (G1, G2, G3, G8, and G9), and in the location where the TEAM Time activity will be held (G6 and G7).

 General → General Signs

G1: Fitness for Life: Elementary School

G2: Wellness Week

G3: Physical Activity Pyramid for Kids

G4: MyPyramid for Kids

G5: Eat Well Wednesday

G6: TEAM Time: Together Everyone Achieves More

G7: Get Fit Friday

G8: Healthy mind, healthy body, healthy heart . . . let's start!

G9: ABCs of Physical Activity

G10: ABCs of Nutrition

Weekly Signs

In addition to the general signs, the DVD includes specific signs that are meant for Wellness Week 4. These signs contain messages that relate to the week's themes. The signs are saved together in one file so you can easily print them all at once. Post the weekly signs in hallways throughout the school.

 Wellness Week 4 → Weekly Signs

Physical Activity Pyramid: Do activities from all the steps!

Eat all of the colors in the pyramid!

If you don't take care of your body, where will you live?

Get off your seat and move your feet!

Get up, get moving, and have some fun. It helps your brain when you get out and run!

Play lots, learn lots!

Play every day, sun or rain. Playing is good for your brain!

Healthy foods help us move! Choose your foods wisely!

Be water wise!

Be sun wise!

If you want to do better than before, make a plan to practice more!

When we play and train, we build our brains!

Combine skills to have some fun!

Energy in (the food we eat) – energy out (how much we move) = a healthy body

To play your best, drink water at every rest!

Personal fitness starts with me!

WEEK 4

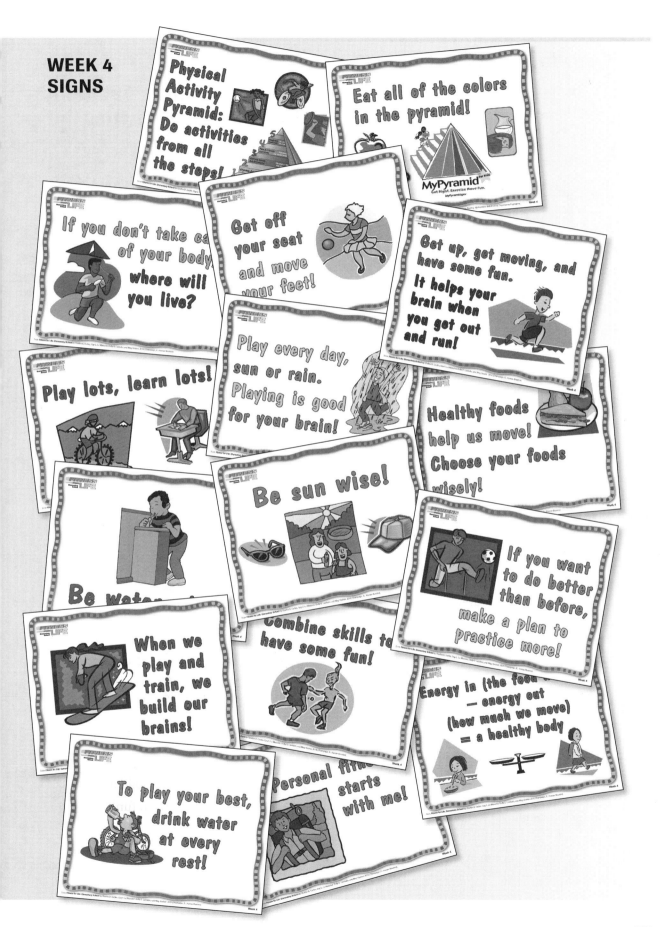

Step 4: Encourage Active Playgrounds

The Active Playgrounds sign file contains signs related to getting kids active while on the playground. The signs are saved together in one file so you can easily print them all at once. Consider saving them in a folder to reuse next year. If possible, have members of the office staff assist you. You may also want to ask students to help with printing and decorating the signs before posting.

Use the following steps to help encourage more active behavior on the playground.

- Print the active playground signs.
- Post the signs near the doors to the playground. Encourage teachers to call attention to these signs.
- Ask staff members or teachers to make some activity equipment available during recess and lunch.
- Create an activity bin that has balls, jump ropes, and so on that can be wheeled out to activity areas.
- Encourage teachers (both classroom and physical education) to help students stay active on the playground by having them do some of the physical activities that they learned during Wellness Week. Encourage activity in tether ball, Four Square, and other sports and activities typically done on your school playground.
- Ask playground supervisors to verbally encourage active play.

The Active Playground signs are listed below. You can see thumbnails of the signs on page 31.

 General → Active Playground Signs

Active play area ahead: Get moving!

You have a green light! Get your body running!

No sitting, no standing! Get active, get moving!

Choose to be active!

Start your engine and get moving now!

Caution: Children moving ahead!

Don't sit, get fit!

Get off your seat and move your feet!

Step 5: Coordinate Eat Well Wednesday Activities

Eat Well Wednesday is devoted to nutrition. Consistent with the weekly theme, the focus of the Eat Well Wednesday activity for Wellness Week 4 is balancing calories and choosing a variety of foods. Make contact with cafeteria workers and other staff ahead of Wellness Week 4 to allow time for the following Eat Well Wednesday activity.

Healthy Choices

This activity encourages children to make healthy food choices every day. Provide a fruit and vegetable selection of foods whose names start with letters from A to Z. Have bottled water as a healthy choice of beverage for the day. Messages for reinforcing the weekly nutrition theme can be found on the table tent signs on the DVD.

Preparation

- Work with staff (ahead of Wellness Week 4) to plan the fruit, vegetable, and water bar. Try to include fruits and vegetables whose names range the alphabet from A to Z.
- Work with the staff to make placards for each of the fruits and vegetables that are available on the food bar so the children can identify what they are eating. If you have ESL students, provide translations in other languages.
- Print the week 4 tent signs from the DVD. They are saved together in one file.

 Wellness Week 4 → Tent Signs

You are what you eat, from your head down to your feet!

Balance energy in (food) with energy out (activity)!

Suggestions

Eat Well Wednesday classroom activities can also be planned. The classroom guides provide

TENT SIGNS

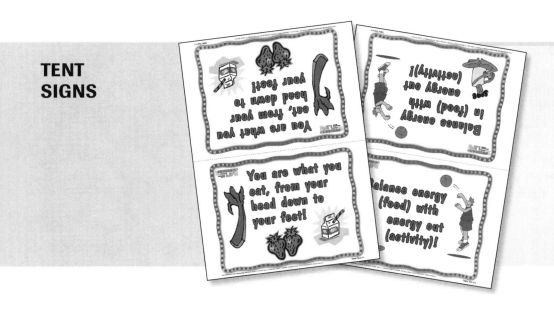

outlines for discussions that promote the Wellness Week 4 nutrition theme.

Cafeteria Signs

The DVD includes general cafeteria signs related to nutrition. The messages and concepts in the signs are discussed in the classroom and in physical education class and are included in video messages. Posting signs will help reinforce these important nutrition and physical activity messages and concepts.

Review the signs, which are saved together in one file in the Cafeteria Signs folder on the DVD, and post as many as desired in the cafeteria during Wellness Week. You can also have students decorate the signs before posting. Consider printing all the cafeteria signs at once and saving them for use next year.

In addition, the General Signs folder contains a file called G10: ABCs of Nutrition, which is a set of 26 signs (one for each letter of the alphabet) that feature nutrition images and messages. During any Wellness Week, you can use the ABCs of Nutrition signs along with, or instead of, the cafeteria signs.

You can see thumbnails of the cafeteria signs on page 33.

 General → General Signs

    G10: ABCs of Nutrition

 General → Cafeteria Signs

    Orange is for grains!

    Green is for veggies!

    Red is for fruits!

    Blue is for milk products!

    Purple is for meat and beans!

    Yellow is for oils. Use them wisely!

    Life is full of choices. Choose healthy foods!

    Be wise. Eat well and exercise!

    Food is fuel for learning and moving. Choose wisely!

    Did you eat the rainbow way today?

    Eat the rainbow way: every color, every day!

    Did you eat your 5 to 9 today?

    Make half your grains whole!

    Protein power! Get strong, live long!

    You are what you eat. Choose wisely!

    Avoid empty calories!

Step 6: Coordinate Get Fit Friday Activities

For Wellness Week 4, the Get Fit Friday activity is TEAM Time 4: Mid Kids Lead. This activity emphasizes the weekly physical activity theme of integration (energy balance) and the concept of TEAM: Together Everyone Achieves More.

WEEK 4

TEAM Time 4: Mid Kids Lead

During the first 10 minutes of school, all students will perform an activity routine that includes a warm-up, an activity called Hawaiian Surfing, and a cool-down. This activity is led by the wellness coordinator and selected third- and fourth-grade students (the mid kids). The goal is to have all the students work together to get some of their 60 minutes of daily activity as recommended by national standards. The theme of the fourth Wellness Week is integration (energy balance), so several types of activity are included in this TEAM Time. Evidence suggests that activity at the beginning of the school day can enhance learning in the classroom (Hillman et al., 2009a; Hillman et al., 2009b; Le Masurier & Corbin, 2006; Ratey, 2008; Smith & Lounsbery, 2009).

TEAM Time 4: Mid Kids Lead uses four tracks on the DVD: an instructional video that shows how one wellness coordinator conducts the activity and three routines (a warm-up, an activity called Hawaiian Surfing, and a cool-down) that you can play when you lead your school. In addition, TEAM Time 4 uses a file of printable resources (a sample outline to follow and the specific exercises in each routine) that are saved together in one file in the following folder.

 Wellness Week 4 → TEAM Time

Messages

- Integration (energy balance)
- TEAM (Together Everyone Achieves More)

Preparation

To prepare for TEAM Time 4: Mid Kids Lead, the following steps are recommended.

- Familiarize yourself with the activity. Watch the instructional video on the DVD, which shows how one wellness coordinator conducts the activity.
- Familiarize yourself with the resources.
- Select some third- and fourth-grade students to help you lead the activity.
- Plan a practice session with the student leaders before the actual TEAM Time 4

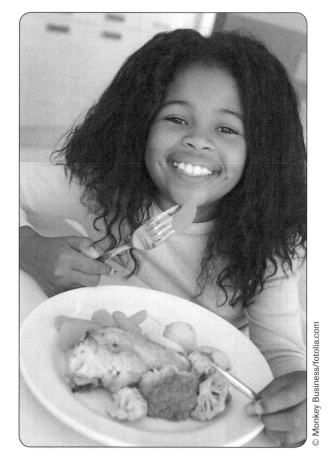

Balancing calories is a part of Wellness Week 4's theme of integration (energy balance).

event. Use the warm-up, Hawaiian Surfing, and cool-down videos on the DVD to learn the movements for each part of the activity. The warm-up and cool-down are the same as those for TEAM Time 2. Help the student leaders learn the movements so that they can help you lead on the day of the event.

- Arrange for a DVD player on the day of the event. If you have a computer and computer projector, you can use them to project a large image.

Activity

- Print a copy of the TEAM Time 4 sample outline from the DVD, or use the one on page 60.
- Set up a DVD player (or computer and computer projector) in the location where TEAM Time will be held.

WEEK 4

- If possible, place a microphone by the DVD speaker so that music for TEAM Time is loud enough for all to hear. Turn the DVD volume up loud.

- You may want to turn the screen of the DVD away from the students so that they focus on watching you and the student leaders rather than everyone watching the routine on the screen.

- Have classroom teachers available to monitor their own classes and encourage active participation.

- After students report to class and roll is taken, teachers lead students to the gym, the multipurpose room, or outside. If the gym or multipurpose room is not big enough to accommodate all the students, you might want to do the activity at the beginning of the day for half the students and again after lunch for the other half.

- Welcome students, give motivational comments, and start the event using procedures similar to those used by the wellness coordinator in the instructional video on the DVD. You can use the sample outline to guide you.

- Make daily announcements or have the principal make daily announcements if there are any.

- Lead the TEAM Time 4 routine with the help of the third- and fourth-grade leaders. Place these leaders around the TEAM Time area so that they are visible to as many children as possible. Encourage students to watch you or your student leaders. If they cannot easily see a leader, encourage them to follow other students who can see a leader.

- Play the warm-up, Hawaiian Surfing, and cool-down videos on the DVD to cue your movements and the movements of student leaders.

- When the routine is finished, congratulate the students. Then dismiss students by calling the names of teachers, who leave with their students as their names are called.

Step 7: Coordinate Special Celebrations

Appendix A of this guide contains complete descriptions of several Wellness Week celebration activities. Encourage teachers and parents to conduct one or more of these celebrations, or if time allows, coordinate the event of your choice. Events from which you may choose include the following:

- Brain Walk
- Family Fun Night
- Fitness-a-Thon
- Fun Run/Walk (could be tied to Halloween or Thanksgiving)
- GYM (Get Yourself Moving) Club
- Fitness Trail
- Pay to Play
- Seasonal events and health observances

Step 8: Assess Responses

Use one or more of the assessment tools to assess student, teacher, and parent responses to the Wellness Week and other school wellness activities. The assessment tools can be found on the DVD or in appendix B (page 92).

 General → Assessments

Classroom Teacher Program Assessment Tool

Physical Education Teacher Program Assessment Tool

Student Video Activity Ratings

Wellness Coordinator Program Assessment Tool

Family Wellness Week Assessment

Family Physical Activity and Nutrition Questionnaire

Analysis Form for Assessments

WEEK 4

SAMPLE OUTLINE

Opening Comments

"Good morning, everybody." (Kids respond with "Good morning." Put a hand up behind your ear to indicate that they are not loud enough.) "I can't hear you. Let's try that again. Good morning, everybody!" (Kids respond with "Good morning!")

"Welcome to TEAM Time. TEAM stands for 'Together Everyone Achieves More.' We are going to do some fun activities as a team to get us ready for the school day. At the end of the routine, we are going to do a chant. Let's practice it so that you are ready when the time comes.

"I'll say it first and then you say it: Stay active, eat well." (Kids respond with "Stay active, eat well.") "Say it again: Stay active, eat well." (Kids respond with "Stay active, eat well.")

"Good job. Now let's get started. I have asked some students to help me lead this TEAM Time activity. Just watch what we do, and try to follow along. Don't worry if you make a mistake. Just do the best that you can."

Activity

Conduct Mid Kids Lead with the warm-up, Hawaiian Surfing, and cool-down videos. During the activity, periodically repeat the following statements to encourage students: "Good job. Nice work. Keep trying, you are getting it. Way to go. Stick with it."

Closing Comments

Have students perform the chant at the end of the routine: "Stay active, eat well."

After the routine, consider using these comments: "Great job! You worked well as a team when doing the TEAM Time activities.

"OK, let's keep working as a team. It's time to go back to your classrooms and remember that Together Everyone Achieves More. Kindergarten students, follow your teacher back to your classroom." (Allow time.) "Now the first-grade students." (Allow time.) "Now the second-grade students." (Allow time. Continue in this manner until all grades are dismissed. Alternatively, you may use a list of teachers' names to let classes know when to begin walking back to their classrooms.)

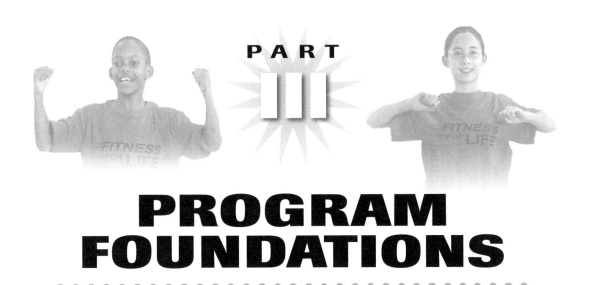

PART III

PROGRAM FOUNDATIONS

Part I of this guide provided a brief overview of the educational foundations used in developing the **Fitness for Life: Elementary School** program. That overview was intentionally brief so you could have quick and early access to the specific information needed for implementing the program. Part III provides additional information for those who want to learn more about the educational foundations on which **FFL: Elementary** is based. Part III is divided into three sections. First, "Links With Academic Achievement" discusses the connections between physical education and other areas of academics. Next, "Educational and Scientific Foundations" delves into the topic of wellness and provides more extensive coverage of physical activity and nutrition guidelines. Finally, "The Obesity Epidemic" presents further details about overweight and obesity among youth.

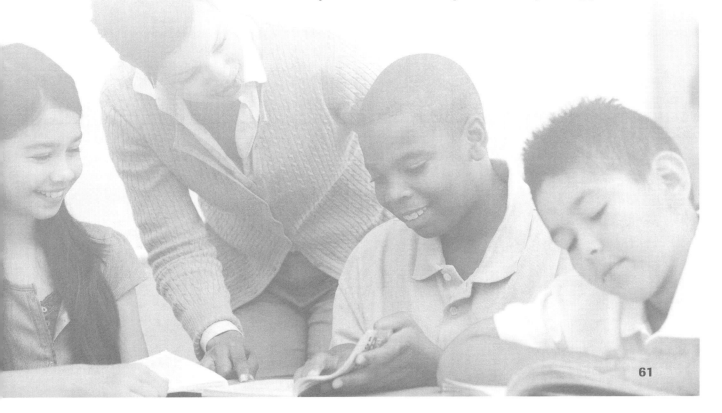

LINKS WITH ACADEMIC ACHIEVEMENT

Fitness for Life Elementary School

The introduction to this guide noted the link between academic achievement and the **Fitness for Life: Elementary School** program. This section explores that link in more depth and specifically discusses the following:

- Physical education and academic achievement
- Physical activity and academic achievement
- Physical fitness and academic achievement
- Physical activity and school success

Physical Education and Academic Achievement

The emphasis on academic testing in recent years has resulted in increased time spent on subjects such as math, science, and language arts. Test scores are important, but the increased time in one subject area in the curriculum often results in decreased time spent on other subjects. The research now clearly indicates that taking time for physical education (20 to 60 minutes) during the day does *not* detract from academic performance in other academics areas—in fact, taking the time for physical education during the day may enhance test scores.

The classic Three Rivers study clearly shows that using time in the school day for physical education *does not* reduce academic performance

in other areas and *does* help children improve fitness and expend calories that help control obesity (Shephard & Trudeau, 2005; Trudeau et al., 1998). Evidence from other studies indicates that increased time in physical education either enhances academic performance (Sallis et al., 1999; Shephard et al., 1994, 1997) or has no negative effect on academic performance (Dwyer et al., 2001; Sallis et al., 1999). Clearly, this research shows that, despite decreased time spent in academics, additional physical activity can improve academic achievement and, at minimum, does not result in lower achievement.

Recent research has shown that students with low test scores who participate in before-school physical education programs improve test scores in a variety of areas. One study, conducted in Naperville, Illinois, is summarized in Ratey's *SPARK: The Revolutionary New Science of Exercise and the Brain* (2008). Students participating in this program improved test scores and academic performance in a variety of areas, including reading and math. More information on the Naperville program is available on the Teacher page of the **FFL: Elementary** Web site (www.fitnessforlife.org).

The bottom line is that reducing the time spent in physical education and activity during the school day is counterproductive. Maintaining a quality physical education program meets important educational goals of many kinds, including important physical education

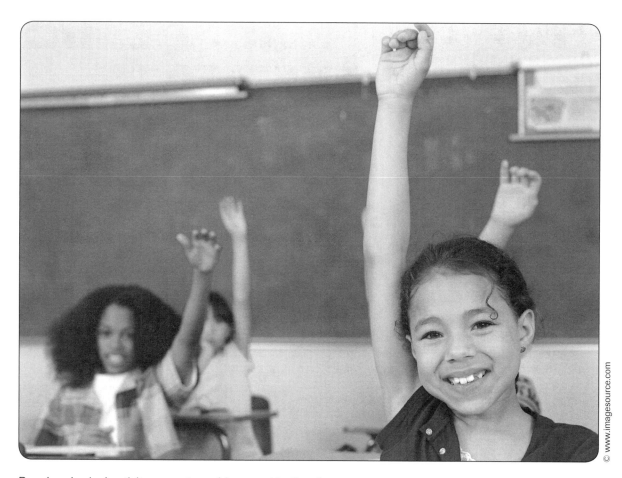

Regular physical activity promotes achievement in the classroom.

goals such as physical fitness achievement, skill development, and an introduction to learning the concepts and principles of activity, to name a few. For more information concerning the link between physical education and academic achievement, see the excellent article by Smith and Lounsbery (2009), "Promoting Physical Education: The Link to Academic Achievement." The complete source information, along with other engaging articles and books, is in the reference section of this book.

Physical Activity and Academic Achievement

A principal reason physical education can positively impact academic achievement is that physical activity improves cognitive function. Sibley and Etnier (2003) performed a meta-analysis of 44 research studies and concluded

that there was a significant positive relationship between physical activity and cognitive functioning in children. Other studies have concluded that 20 to 50 minutes of physical activity positively affects cognitive function (20 minutes, Sibley, Etnier, Pangrazi, & Le Masurier, 2006; 30 minutes, McNaughten & Gabbard, 1993; and 50 minutes, Gabbard & Barton, 1979).

The book *SPARK: The Revolutionary New Science of Exercise and the Brain* (2008), by Harvard professor John Ratey, has stimulated interest in the study of exercise and brain function. In his book, Ratey extols the benefits of physical activity on brain functioning and cognitive performance. In addition to discussing the relationship between physical education and academic achievement, he includes chapters on exercise and its relationship to attention disorders, exercise and brain cells, stress, and anxiety reduction, all relevant directly or indirectly to academic performance.

Physical Fitness and Academic Achievement

Several states conduct regular physical fitness testing of their youth. Using data from statewide testing, California was among the first to study the relationship between fitness test scores as measured by Fitnessgram (a national youth fitness test) and scores on statewide achievement tests (Ernst, Corbin, Beighle, & Pangrazi, 2006). Reports published by the California Department of Education (2003, 2005) show a positive relationship between fitness scores and academic achievement and an inverse relationship between academic achievement and BMI (body mass index, the ratio of fat to overall body mass, frequently used as a measure of a healthy weight). Fit children had higher academic scores than less fit children, and children with higher BMI scores had lower academic scores than children with lower BMIs. The California results are consistent with results reported by Castelli, Hillman, Buck, and Erwin (2006) that showed aerobic capacity (cardiovascular fitness) scores are positively related with math and reading scores, and BMI scores are inversely associated with math and reading scores.

A large-scale study of the fitness of Texas youth also showed that fitness (Fitnessgram test scores) is positively associated with academic test scores, and that BMI scores are negatively associated with academic performance. In addition, the Texas study showed that the relationship between fitness and academic scores was present even when school size, school socioeconomic status, or minority status were considered. More information concerning the Texas study is available at www.ourkidshealth.org. Studies in Massachusetts (Chomitz et al., 2009) and New York City yielded similar findings. The New York City study is available at http://schools.nyc.gov/Offices/mediarelations/NewsandSpeeches/2009-2010/20090713_fitness_report.htm.

It is important to note that the studies cited in this section show correlations only. They clearly establish that there is a relationship between fitness and academic test scores, but further research is necessary to determine causality (e.g., does fitness cause academic success or does academic success lead to fitness?). However, the studies cited in earlier sections of this chapter strongly suggest that physical activity that promotes physical fitness can be beneficial to the academic performance of children.

Physical Activity and School Success

Regular attendance at school is not a direct indicator of school success. However, most would agree that missing school is not beneficial to performance in school. The physical fitness studies of Texas youth show that fit youth are absent from school less often than unfit youth. Further, the data show that youth who are fit are less likely than unfit youth to be involved in negative school incidents such as fighting and disruptive behavior. More information is available at www.ourkidshealth.org.

Summary

The preponderance of evidence indicates that physical activity during the school day benefits youth in many ways. Time taken for activity breaks such as those planned for Wellness Week help children to get fit, meet national activity goals, and be more successful academically.

EDUCATIONAL AND SCIENTIFIC FOUNDATIONS

Fitness for Life Elementary School

The introduction to this guide provided an overview of the educational and scientific foundations for the **Fitness for Life: Elementary School** program. This section provides additional details.

Wellness Foundations

According to the Child Nutrition and WIC (Women, Infants and Children) Reauthorization Act (Public Law 108-265) passed by Congress in 2004, all states, school districts, and schools receiving funding for school lunch programs must have a policy (or plan) designed to encourage total school wellness. A document describing the act is available at the USDA Web site listed in the resources section at the end of this book. Central to a sound wellness policy is the notion that the primary mission of schools is to promote optimal learning for all children, and this cannot be achieved if students are not fit and healthy.

Implementing **FFL: Elementary** will help your school comply with the act. The following are some components of a sound school wellness policy, based on information from the United States Department of Agriculture (USDA) (www.usda.gov/wps/portal/usdahome) and other organizations such as Action for Healthy Kids (www.actionforhealthykids.org).

According to the USDA, the following should be present in a sound wellness program:

- Students are provided with opportunities for physical activity in the classroom, in physical education, before school, at recess, and after school.
- Students receive nutrition education in the classroom, in physical education, and in the cafeteria.
- Students are provided with nutrition, physical activity, and other wellness messages in the classroom and throughout the school.
- Healthy eating is promoted through healthy meals at school and healthy snacks at school.
- Nutrition and physical activity are integrated into the health education and core curriculum areas (e.g., math, science, language arts).
- Information (including messages) is consistent throughout the school.
- The school wellness policy is based on national standards for nutrition, physical activity, and physical education.
- Opportunities for in-service training and employee wellness are available to all school employees (teachers, administration, food service, and other staff) to aid

in implementation of school wellness policy.

- A system of evaluation is in place to assess program effectiveness.

Action for Healthy Kids is a national non-profit organization dedicated to addressing the epidemic of overweight, undernourished, and sedentary youth by focusing on changes in schools. This organization works throughout the United States to improve children's nutrition and increase physical activity, and by doing so, help them get more from their education (www.actionforhealthykids.org). The Action for Healthy Kids Web site has an excellent Wellness Policy Tool that can be used online to help you plan a school wellness program. In addition, the Web site includes links to state wellness programs and examples of wellness plans developed for many different schools. Other resources, such as evaluations tools, are also provided.

Physical Activity Pyramid for Kids

The Physical Activity Pyramid for Kids (PA Pyramid) provides a model for the various types of physical activities that promote health and fitness among youth. It was created by Charles B. Corbin and is used in all **Fitness for Life** programs, in the Fitnessgram program, and (with permission) by other programs such as Physical Best.

There are two versions of the PA Pyramid, one for kids and one for teens. **FFL: Elementary** uses the pyramid developed specifically for kids (see figure 3.1).

Five Steps

In **FFL: Elementary** both physical activity and nutrition are emphasized. MyPyramid, as presented earlier, shows steps on the left side that represent physical activity. The PA Pyramid is a visual representation of these steps. Each step represents a different type of physical activity. In full-color versions of the PA Pyramid, each of the five steps of the pyramid is presented in a color that is also used in MyPyramid.

Step 1: Moderate Physical Activity

Moderate physical activity is depicted as the first step in the PA Pyramid because it is the most common type of physical activity (activities equal in intensity to brisk walking) performed by most Americans. Moderate activities include lifestyle activities, such as working in the yard or walking to the store. For children it includes moderate-intensity play, walking to school, doing chores at home, and other similar activities. Moderate activity is recommended daily for children. The first Wellness Week focuses on moderate physical activity. In the color version of the PA Pyramid, the first step is shown in orange, the same color as used for grains in MyPyramid. Grains are a major source of energy, and moderate activity is a major type of activity for most people, including children.

Steps 2 and 3: Vigorous Activities

Vigorous aerobic activities (such as jogging and aerobic dance) are on the second step in the PA Pyramid and are shown in the color green, the same as vegetables in MyPyramid. Vigorous sports and recreation (such as tennis, soccer, hiking, and biking) are on the third step in the pyramid and are shown in the color red, the same color used for fruits in MyPyramid. These activities are considered to be vigorous because they are of higher intensity (e.g., elevate the breathing and heart rates) than moderate-intensity activities. Vigorous activities should be included in much of the activity that children perform. In fact, national guidelines recommend that some of the 60 minutes of activity each day should be vigorous in nature. At a minimum, children should perform vigorous activity at least three days a week. Vigorous physical activity is the focus of the second Wellness Week.

Step 4: Muscle Fitness Exercises

The fourth step of the PA Pyramid, muscle fitness exercise, is shown in blue, the same color used for milk in MyPyramid. Muscle fitness exercise for children includes doing calisthenics, such as push-ups and curl-ups, performing gymnastics stunts, doing exercises with elastic

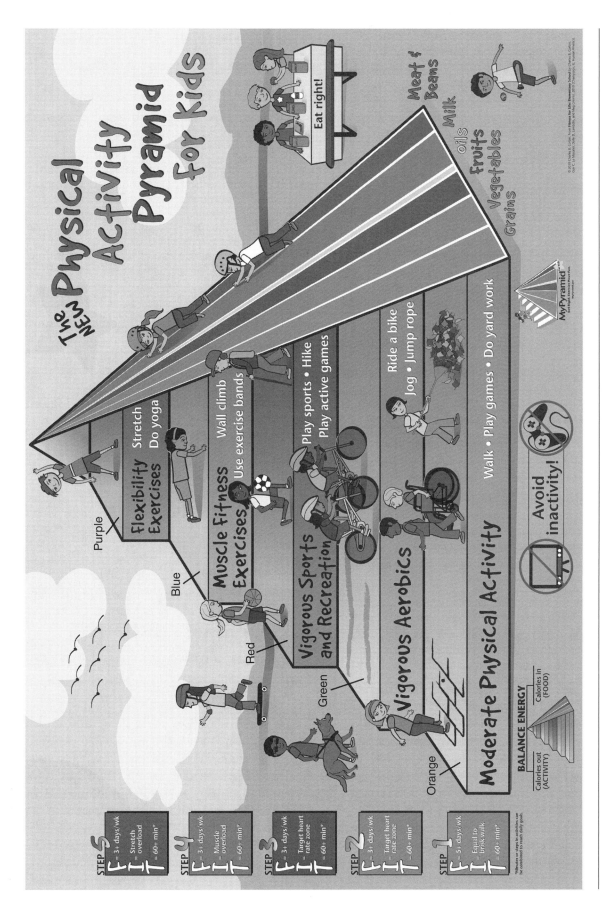

Figure 3.1 Children can meet national physical activity guidelines by doing activities from the five levels of the Physical Activity Pyramid for Kids.

©2010 Charles B. Corbin

bands, and any other activities that overload the large muscles of the body. Muscle fitness exercises also stress the long bones of the body and are important to bone development in youth. National guidelines recommend participation in muscle fitness exercises and activities at least two or three days a week. Muscle fitness exercises are highlighted in the third Wellness Week.

Step 5: Flexibility Exercises

The fifth step of the PA Pyramid includes exercises that build flexibility (e.g., stretching exercises and movements requiring a large range of motion); this step is shown in purple, the same color used for meat and beans in MyPyramid. Regular stretching exercises and activities for developing flexibility should be performed at least three days a week and as frequently as every day. To build flexibility, muscles and tendons must be stretched for longer periods of time than are normal, in activities such as gymnastics, yoga, and stretching exercises (e.g., zipper, back saver sit-and-reach). Like muscle fitness exercises, flexibility exercises are highlighted in the third Wellness Week.

Around the Pyramid

Inactivity and sedentary living are depicted below the PA Pyramid. National guidelines suggest that long periods of inactivity (two hours or more) should be avoided. Of course, some inactivity is important, such as regular sleep at night and doing homework. However, excess TV and the use of computer games take time that reduces activity levels.

At the right side of the PA Pyramid, the color bands of MyPyramid are shown. This demonstrates that the PA Pyramid and MyPyramid are two sides of the same pyramid. When considered from one angle, the PA Pyramid is more prominent, and when considered from a different angle, MyPyramid is more prominent.

The fourth Wellness Week focuses on energy balance. The goal is to expend calories in any form of physical activity from the PA Pyramid (avoiding sedentary living) and balancing the calories expended in activity with calories consumed in food from MyPyramid. Beneath the

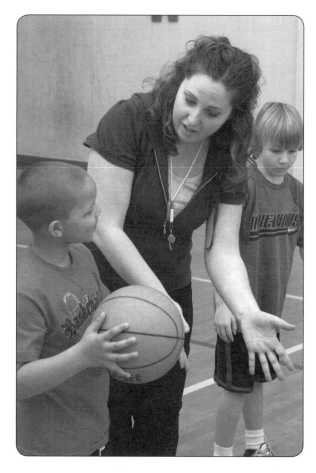

Fitness for Life: Elementary School is based on national standards for physical education and other subject matter areas.

PA Pyramid, a balance scale depicts the need for energy balance to maintain a healthy weight.

National (USDHHS) Physical Activity Guidelines

Over the years there have been many different sets of guidelines for physical activity. Although adult physical activity guidelines have been available for some time, it was not until 1998 that guidelines specifically for children were developed (NASPE, 1998). In 2004 the guidelines were revised (NASPE, 2004b). The CDC developed separate but similar guidelines in 2005 (Strong et al., 2005). In the fall of 2008 the United States Department of Health and Human Services (USDHHS) developed the first set of national guidelines for people of all ages (USDHHS, 2008). A brief summary of the guidelines was provided in the Program Introduction (page 11). A more complete description of the guidelines for children from the comprehensive guidelines for people of all ages is presented below; go to www.health.gov/paguidelines/ for more detail.

Following is the activity recommended each week:

- Perform physical activity 60 minutes (or more) each day.

- Activity can be from any of the first three steps of the PA Pyramid (for kids).

- Moderate activity is activity equal in intensity to brisk walking (step 1 of the pyramid). For children this could include walking to school, doing yard work at home, or moderate play. Riding a bicycle at a slow speed also qualifies as moderate activity.

- Moderate activity should be done on most or all days of the week.

- Vigorous activity is activity that elevates the heart rate into the target zone. It includes activities from the second and third steps of the PA Pyramid. This includes vigorous sports, vigorous recreation and play, and vigorous aerobic activities such as jogging and aerobic dance.

- Vigorous activity should be performed at least three days per week.

- Stretching and muscle fitness activities that build muscles and bones should be performed at least three days per week.

- For children, activity need not be continuous as it is for adults—the activity can be performed intermittently, but the focus should be on more activity than rest over a given period of time.

National Physical Education Curriculum Standards

The National Association for Sport and Physical Education (NASPE, 2004a) identified standards for curriculum in physical education that have been used by 48 of the 50 states in developing state standards and physical education curriculum. These standards define the content needed to help individuals have the knowledge, skills, and confidence to enjoy a lifetime of healthy physical activity. There are six major standards on which **FFL: Elementary** is based:

A physically educated person be able to do the following:

- Demonstrate competency in motor skills and movement patterns needed to perform a variety of physical activities (standard 1).

- Demonstrate understanding of movement concepts, principles, strategies, and tactics as they apply to the learning and performance of physical activities (standard 2).

- Participate regularly in physical activity (standard 3).

- Achieve and maintain a health-enhancing level of physical fitness (standard 4).

- Exhibit responsible personal and social behavior that respects self and others in physical activity settings (standard 5).

- Value physical activity for health, enjoyment, challenge, self-expression, and/or social interaction.

From National Association for Sport and Physical Education. (2004). *Moving into the future: National standards for physical education.* 2nd ed. Reston, VA: Author.

The performance standards for each grade level (K-2, 3-5, 6) are included in appendix D.

National Standards for Math, Language Arts, and Science

In addition to the national physical education curriculum standards (NASPE), standards for other subject matter were also considered. The following are Web addresses for finding more information about standards in a variety of subject areas:

National Math Standards (National Council of Teachers of Mathematics)

Focal points by grade are available at www.nctm.org/standards/.

National Social Studies Standards

A draft copy is available at www.socialstudies. org/standards/taskforce/fall2008draft.

National Language Arts Standards (National Council of Teachers of English)

The standards are available for purchase at www1.ncte.org/store/books/bestsellers/105977. htm?source=gs.

National Science Standards

- www.nsta.org/publications/nses.aspx
- www.educationworld.com/standards/ national/toc/index.shtml#science

National Nutrition Standards

As noted in the introduction, nutrition guidelines from the United States Department of Agriculture (USDA) provide the basis for the nutrition information in **FFL: Elementary**. Every five years a committee of the USDA revises the National Nutrition Guidelines. The most recent revision was in 2005 at which time MyPyramid was developed and the focus shifted from servings to cups. In addition, the 2005 guidelines made the following recommendations.

- Increase consumption from the dairy group. Children ages 2 to 8 should consume 2 cups per day (e.g., fat-free or low-fat milk or equivalent milk products). Children 9 and older should consume 3 cups per day.
- Consume whole-grain products often.
- Choose and prepare foods and beverages with little added sugar or other sugar-based sweeteners.
- Reduce consumption of sugar- and starch-containing foods.
- Limit total fat intake. Children ages 4 to 18 should consume no more than 35 percent of diet as fat.
- Most dietary fat should come from foods containing polyunsaturated or monounsaturated fats (e.g., fish, nuts, canola oil).

MyPyramid for Kids (www.fns.usda.gov/tn/ kids-pyramid.html) was briefly described in the introduction. MyPyramid for Kids (figure 3.2) is an adaptation of MyPyramid, a tool for guiding adult Americans to eat well. MyPyramid for Kids is much more than just a food guide. It has many additional resources, including worksheets, posters, and a Web tool for children.

The following are brief descriptions of each food category, as adapted from MyPyramid.

- Orange represents grains. Any food made from wheat, rice, oats, cornmeal, barley, or another cereal grain is a grain product. Bread, pasta, oatmeal, breakfast cereals, tortillas, and grits are examples of grain products.
- Green represents vegetables. Any vegetable or 100-percent vegetable juice counts as a member of the vegetable group. Vegetables may be raw or cooked; fresh, frozen, canned, or dried or dehydrated; and may be whole, cut up, or mashed.
- Red represents fruits. Any fruit or 100-percent fruit juice counts as part of the fruit group. Fruits may be fresh, canned, frozen, or dried, and may be whole, cut up, or pureed.
- Blue represents milk. All fluid milk products and many foods made from milk are considered part of this food group. Foods made from milk that retain their calcium content are part of the group, while foods made from milk that have little to no calcium, such as cream cheese, cream, and butter, are not. Most milk group choices should be fat-free or low-fat.
- Purple represents meat and beans. All foods made from meat, poultry, fish, dry beans or peas, eggs, nuts, and seeds are considered part of this group. Dry beans and peas are part of this group as well as the vegetable group.
- Yellow represents oils. Oils are fats that are liquid at room temperature, like the vegetable oils used in cooking. Oils come from many different plants and from fish.

The steps on the side of MyPyramid represent the various forms of physical activity that are

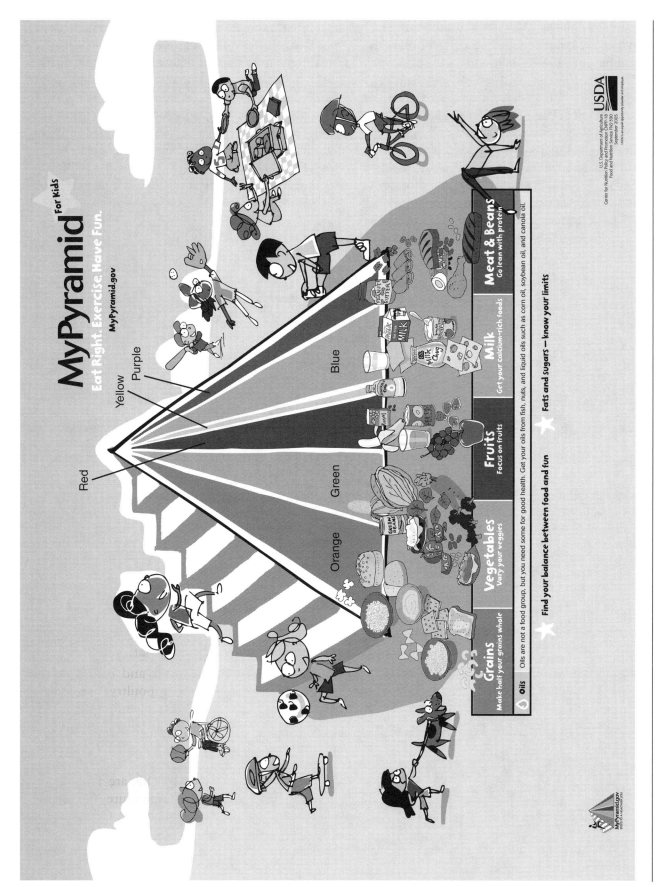

Figure 3.2   Fitness for Life: Elementary School helps children learn about MyPyramid and sound nutrition.

Adapted from U.S. Department of Agriculture.

also depicted in the PA Pyramid. Both foods and activities are color coded. The USDA nutrition guidelines emphasize the importance of physical activity, together with sound nutrition, in promoting health and wellness. A balance of calories taken in (from MyPyramid) and calories expended (PA Pyramid) is the key.

Additional nutrition standards adapted from *Model Guidelines for Health and Wellness*, a booklet published by nine major health-related organizations, were considered in the development of **FFL: Elementary**. The model guidelines call for increased nutrition education, including integration in other subject areas such as physical education, science, social studies, and literature. The guidelines also call for an improved food environment in the school (e. g., cafeteria environment, scheduling of lunch and breakfast) and changes in food service operations (e.g., food service personnel, menus, community involvement). The booklet is available on the DVD in this guide and was created by the Council for Corporate and School Partnerships (sponsored by The Coca-Cola Company).

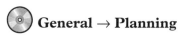 **General → Planning**

THE OBESITY EPIDEMIC

Fitness for Life
Elementary School

In the introduction and in the Executive Summary, we described one of the benefits of **Fitness for Life: Elementary School** as helping to prevent obesity by increasing physical activity and promoting healthy eating. In this section, additional information about the obesity epidemic is provided. This additional information will be useful when talking with parents and school staff members. This information is not included in the other **FFL: Elementary** books, and for this reason you may choose to lend this guide to other teachers and staff members who want to learn more.

The Facts About Youth Overweight and Obesity

The word *epidemic* refers to the occurrence of a disease that exceeds what would normally be expected. Whether or not obesity is considered a disease, and there is debate about that, the incidence of obesity in our culture is exceptionally high—much greater than would be expected. Recent evidence indicates that 66 percent of Americans over the age of 20 are overweight or obese. The most recent data indicate that 15 to 17 percent of youth are obese (this varies with age) and more than 30 percent are overweight. The prevalence of overweight or obese children and adolescents has tripled since these data were first collected in the 1980s. Energy balance (calories consumed equals calories expended)

is critical to maintaining a healthy body weight. Eating well and being active, as promoted in **FFL: Elementary,** are critical in the fight to reduce obesity in children. Further, extra weight and obesity are linked to many diseases of sedentary lifestyles and poor nutrition, including diabetes, coronary heart disease, and hypertension. Chronic diseases such as type 2 diabetes, formerly considered to be adult conditions, are now seen in children and adolescents.

A person is considered overweight when he has more body weight (especially body fat) than is desirable for good health. Obesity occurs when the body weight is extremely high, and the health risk is especially exaggerated. Experts agree that the best methods for assessing whether one is overweight involve the use of lab tests that require special equipment and require assessment by experts. Some examples include underwater weighing and electric impedance machines, among others. Height–weight measurements, body mass index (BMI), and skinfold measurements are common field tests used to screen for overweight or obese children. They can be performed on large numbers of people without a lot of equipment. They do require some training to be used effectively but not as much as is required for lab tests.

In **FFL: Elementary**, fitness assessments from the Fitnessgram are used. In addition, the body mass index (BMI) is used in one of the **FFL: Elementary** activities for grades 3 to 6. The BMI uses height and weight in a special formula to calculate body mass index. The BMI is considered by most experts to be better than height–weight measures for screening for excessive weight or obesity, although, like height–weight measures, the BMI will misclassify some people as overweight or obese, including those high in bone or muscle mass. The BMI (and height–weight measures) can also be useful for screening for people with eating disorders. Because of possible errors in measurement, the BMI is typically used as a screening tool. Those who have exceptionally high or low BMIs may be advised to see a doctor, especially if scores have previously been in a range considered to be more healthy. Tracking to identify changes is important. The American Academy of Pediatrics encourages pediatricians and parents to track the BMI of children over time.

Assessment Standards

Fitnessgram, a national physical fitness test for youth, offers both skinfold measurements and the BMI for screening youth for excess weight and obesity. Because **FFL: Elementary** uses the BMI, rather than the other techniques, only BMI standards are discussed here. Those interested in knowing more about skinfold measurements and healthy fitness zone standards are referred to www.fitnessgram.net (click on Reference Guide and then Fitnessgram Parent Overview (download); the PDF document provides information about skinfold measurements and other body composition assessments on pages 11-19).

The formula for calculating BMI using imperial measurements:

BMI = weight (lb) / [height (in)]^2 × 703

Formula for calculating BMI using metric measurements:

BMI = weight (kg) / [height (m)]^2

In adults, a BMI of 25 to 29.9 is considered overweight and a BMI of 30 and above is considered obese. A BMI calculator is available on the Web (http://apps.nccd.cdc.gov/dnpabmi/) to help you determine whether children and adolescents are overweight or obese. Also, the standards for the healthy fitness zone for

different children of different ages and sexes are available at www.fitnessgram.net (click on Reference Guide and then Fitnessgram Healthy Fitness Zone Standards). Additional information on BMI is available at www.cdc.gov/obesity/childhood/defining.htm.

Risks of Overweight and Obesity in Youth

Being overweight or obese can have serious physical consequences for children and adolescents as well as adults. It is well known that overweight and obese children are more likely to have risk factors associated with cardiovascular disease such as high blood pressure, high cholesterol, and type 2 diabetes. Research also suggests that overweight and obese children are on track for a lifetime of these problems because obese children and adolescents are likely to become obese as adults (Serdula et al., 1993; Whitaker et al., 1997). There is also the potential for negative psychosocial consequences for obese children and adolescents including social discrimination (not a direct problem of obesity, but an unfortunate reality in society), low self-esteem, and depression.

Preventing Overweight and Obesity

When children struggle in math, reading, or writing, there are supports to help them get back on track. There should be help for children struggling with their weight as well. Schools need to become environments that support physical activity and healthy nutrition for all children. Schools need to have programs in place to start and keep students on a healthy lifestyle track. Establishing and implementing a school wellness policy is a great first step, but schools need to create a culture of healthy living that reaches out to parents and community support networks (for instance, recreation centers, physical activity clubs, and local champions of physical activity and nutrition). In order to keep students on a healthy lifestyle track, physical activity and healthy nutrition need to

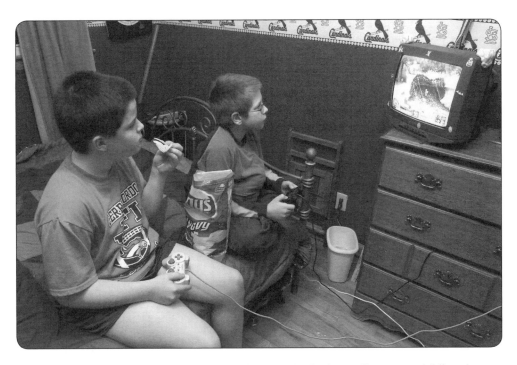

Sedentary living and excessive calorie intake are principal contributors to childhood obesity.

be reinforced throughout the school year. The Wellness Week approach of **FFL: Elementary** is one practical and feasible approach to creating a wellness policy for your school, establishing a healthy lifestyle culture, and combating excess weight and obesity.

Screening for Eating Disorders

Much attention is given to excess weight and obesity. Less attention is given to those who are low in body weight (and fat). Of special con-

cern are conditions such as anorexia nervosa and bulimia. These conditions, most common among teen girls, may have their beginnings in elementary school. Care should be taken, when taking body measurements and when discussing being overweight or obese, not to overdramatize the conditions. Confidentiality in assessment is essential. Screening programs that are caring and educational can help both those high and low in body weight. Youth with screening assessments indicating low weight, especially when those scores have recently changed dramatically, may be referred to a health care professional.

APPENDIX A

Celebration Activities

The **Fitness for Life: Elementary School** program promotes regular physical activity and sound nutrition in four Wellness Weeks throughout the year. As time allows, you, as the wellness coordinator, may choose to conduct some special celebration activities. This appendix presents guidelines for selecting and conducting celebration activities, followed by eight possible types of activities from which to choose. The DVD includes printable resources for many of the activities, along with a blank certificate that you can print and customize for use with your own activities and events.

Early in the School Year

- Choose a celebration activity from this appendix (for each Wellness Week).
- Read the celebration description and make sure it is a good fit for your school community.
- Well ahead of time, designate a date and a location. Mark it on your school or district calendar.
- Start recruiting parent volunteers (if needed).
- Share plans with fellow staff members during a staff meeting and follow up with a written description. Make sure everyone knows his or her role and responsibility during the week.

One Week Before the Activity

- Confirm specific dates and times for the Wellness Week celebration event.
- Contact your local media and tell them about Wellness Week and invite them to your celebration event.

- Begin daily announcements.
- Send fliers and letters to student homes promoting the Wellness Week and the celebration event.
- Have teachers begin promoting the celebration event in their classrooms.
- Recruit your support staff (janitors, cooks, administrative assistants, librarians, and counselors) to participate.
- Encourage your parent-teacher organization and student government committee to help promote the event.
- Encourage your PTA or PTO to participate.
- If you are giving out certificates or need printed materials for participants, now would be the time to send them to the printer.

During Wellness Week

- Contact the volunteers (if needed), assign them individual duties, and ask them to arrive 30 minutes before the event.
- Finalize your event logistics: Use a checklist to determine if you have everything you'll need.
- Plan music, and if you're using a sound system, make sure it works.
- Finalize your backup plan (inclement weather plan).
- Continue daily announcements about Wellness Week and the celebration event.
- When the whole school begins celebrating Wellness Week, promote physical activity, using themes and video messages.

- Contact your local media and remind them of the date, time, and location of your celebration event.
- Assign someone to take pictures.

The Day of the Activity

- Set up everything you'll need.
- Check in volunteers, if any, and remind them of their assigned duties.
- Check music and sound system.
- Remind classroom teachers of the event.
- Decorate the site to make your event as festive as possible.
- Greet participants with lots of fanfare, music, and announcements; remember it's a celebration!
- Explain the event procedures either through an all-school announcement or PA announcement to kick off the event.
- End with a group celebration reiterating the Wellness Week theme.

After the Activity

- Reflect on the event and gather input from other teachers and volunteers to help make your next event even better.
- Write thank-you notes to volunteers.
- Write a wrap-up of the event, with pictures, for the school newsletter and Web site.
- Start planning your next event!
- Begin promoting the next Wellness Week and event.

Celebration Activity 1: Brain Walk

Description

The Brain Walk can be held before schoolwide or classroom tests or exams. Students walk through the school or on the playground before tests. Research suggests that doing physical activity before school and during school can help student achievement in the classroom. Activity may also be beneficial before tests or exams, helping students relax and reducing test anxiety (Hillman et al., 2009a; Hillman et al., 2009b;

Smith & Lounsbery, 2009). As the wellness coordinator, you may want to organize a Brain Walk before schoolwide exams or encourage classroom teachers to use the activity.

Purpose

To help students relax before tests or exams and to improve test performance

Planning

Determine when tests are to be given. The walk can be conducted by a single class or many classes if testing is for more than one group. Print and post the Brain Walk sign and the arrow signs. Arrange for music.

 General → Celebrations

CA1 Brain Walk

Equipment

- School signs
- CD player if music is used
- The same music as used for TEAM Time 1: School Walk (see page 34)

Directions

The procedures for the Brain Walk are the same as for the TEAM Time activity for Wellness Week 1. Print the Brain Walk sign and as many arrow signs as you need. Post the arrow signs in the halls or on the playground to designate the path of the walk.

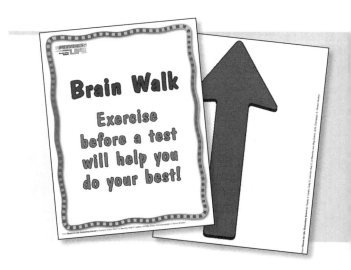

Brain Walk

Exercise before a test will help you do your best!

★ **teacher tip** • • •
Before conducting the Brain Walk, watch the DVD video for TEAM Time 1: School Walk to refresh your memory of this type of activity. The instructional video shows how a wellness coordinator might conduct the School Walk, and the music track provides music for you to use during the activity.

The length of the walk can vary from 5 to 10 minutes. If all students in the school do the Brain Walk, play music on the school sound system as students and teachers walk through the halls or on the playground. Use the same music that was used for the TEAM Time 1: School Walk activity (see page 34).

Celebration Activity 2: Family Fun Night

Description

An organized school event where students and families participate in a variety of physical activities that encourage families to play together. Due to space limitations, these are usually organized around grade levels or certain classrooms.

Purpose

To give students an opportunity to be active, and to teach the parents how to be active with their children

Planning

- Decide which grade level(s) will participate in FFL Family Fun Night.

- Designate a date, time, and place. This is usually an evening event, held in the gym, that lasts about an hour.

- Make a flier to send home announcing the FFL Family Fun Night. You can print and use the FFL Family Fun Night flier on the DVD.

- Plan your evening using activities from the FFL physical education lessons or the classroom guide (see page 82 for an example). Include TEAM Time activities as well.

- Determine the equipment you will need.

- Make sure you have access to a PA system.

- Determine the music you will need.

- Plan to use a projector to show the FFL DVDs on the wall where everyone can see them.

- Decide whether you will provide water and snacks afterwards.

- Decide whether you will give out FFL Family Fun Night certificates of appreciation. You can use the blank certificate template supplied on the DVD.

 General → Celebrations

Blank certificate

CA2 Family Fun Night

Equipment

The equipment will vary depending on the activities selected. For TEAM Time activities,

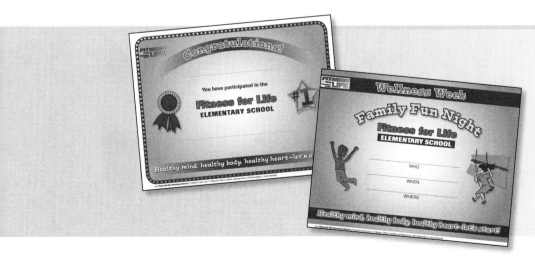

SAMPLE FAMILY FUN NIGHT PLAN

Level: First and Second Grade

Date: Wednesday, May 15

Time: 6:30 – 7:30 pm

Where: In the Independence Elementary School Gymnasium

What: Fitness for Life: Elementary School Family Fun Night. Please come dressed to move. Wear your tennis shoes!

1. Welcome and Introductions (myself, the physical education curriculum, and the **FFL: Elementary** program) Message: "Get off your seat and move your feet!"

2. TEAM Time Routine (warm-up, Colors activity, cool-down from TEAM Time 2: Big Kids Lead).

3. Instant Activities
   - Move and Freeze
   - Athletes in Motion
   - Warm It Up
   - Active Every Day
   - Healthy Body Tag

4. Fitness Activities
   - Animal Antics
   - Grab Bag
   - Move Your Body

5. Skill Adventure
   - CYIM Fit
   - La Raspa
   - Tossing and Catching Skills
   - Jumping for Joy
   - Sport Centers

6. Culminating Activity
   - Fruits and Veggies Tag
   - Cardio Caper
   - Cool It Down

7. Closure, discussion, and questions and answers. Be sure to thank everyone for coming and participating. (And don't forget to acknowledge and thank your volunteers.)

Remember to get off your seat and move your feet!

the DVD that comes with this book and a DVD player will be required.

Directions

- Develop your flier and send it home.
- Make sure the classroom teachers involved know about your event. Ideally, they will help plan, attend, and participate. Have them remind their students of the event throughout the week and especially on the day it is held.
- Plan your event. Select the activities you will do and the messages you will focus on.

Variations

You can add some of your own favorite activities or select some from *Physical Best Activity Guide: Elementary Level* (NASPE, 2004c).

Celebration Activity 3: Fitness-a-Thon

Description

Students participate in a variety of physical activities that are distributed around the play area. At each center, students play or practice a particular physical activity. The centers are monitored by teachers, who travel with their class, from center to center. This activity is very much like a field day.

Purpose

To give students another opportunity to be active

Planning

- Decide on the day and time the Fitness-a-Thon celebration will be held.
- Determine if the entire school will participate or if it will be split into smaller groups.
- Choose the centers.
- Select volunteers, if any (for instance, classroom teachers or older students).
- Make a list of needed equipment.
- Determine length of time participants should stay at each center. (Fifteen minutes should be plenty of time.)

Equipment

Center equipment will depend on the activities selected.

- Air horn or whistle to designate when to change
- Signs and instructions for centers (created by you)
- Information for classroom teachers, including list of centers, rotation schedule, and general rules and guidelines (created by you)

Directions

- Designate a starting activity for each class. Give the classroom teacher a rotation schedule.
- Set up your stations, including equipment, designate them with a sign, and provide instructions, if needed.
- At the designated time all classes will proceed to the field, find their first activity, and begin participating. When the signal sounds, have each class clean up the center and rotate to the next activity.
- Continue this way until everyone has finished. Sixty to ninety minutes is plenty of time.

Possible Centers and Activities

Additional details on these activities are available in the *Physical Education Lesson Plans*.

- Fruits and Veggies Tag
- Cardio Caper
- Jumping for Joy
- Move and Freeze
- Grab Bag
- PACER Practice

teacher tip • • •
   Use low organized games and activities. Let the classroom teachers help!

- Muscle Builder Tag
- Move and Freeze
- What's the Catch?
- Safety Scramble
- Pirate Fitness
- Power Yoga
- Sport Centers
- Olympic Athlete Workout

Variations

Turn it into a playground play day instead, and have your older students teach your younger students the playground games and rules.

Celebration Activity 4: Fun Run/Walk

Description

Everyone will be walking or jogging simultaneously. Designate a course outside on the playground or field for walking and jogging. Everyone joins in by jogging or walking around the designated area for a designated amount of time. This can also be accomplished by grade level, individual classes, or physical education classes. This activity is similar to the Brain Walk and the TEAM Time activity for Wellness Week 1 except that it is done outside and can include parents and other family members as well as students. Jogging or running is optional.

Purpose

This activity gets all students active in walking, running, and jogging. When possible, an additional purpose is to get children active with their parents and other family members.

Planning

- Decide where to hold this event.
- Decide if it is feasible to do with the whole school or it should be split into smaller groups.

- Determine if there should be two separate sites or two separate times.
- Decide if you will stay on campus or go out into the community.
- Decide on the length of the event.
- Recruit volunteers, if they are needed.
- Plan the marking of the designated area.
- Address bathroom logistics.
- Decide if you will give out certificates or completion ribbons.
- Determine if you will use music and, if so, need the PA system.

Equipment

- Traffic cones
- Field paint
- Boat horn or whistle
- PA system
- FFL Fun Run Certificate

💿 **General → Celebrations**

CA4 Fun Run-Walk

Directions

- Designate an area, race route, or track for the event with cones or marking paint.
- At the designated time teachers will bring their students to the designated area and begin walking or jogging.
- When the time is up, have a boat horn, whistle, or bell to sound wildly to signify that the event is over.

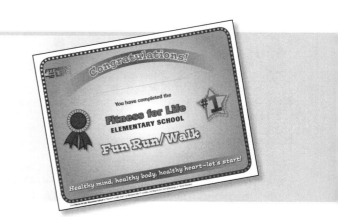

⭐ **teacher tip** • • •
Let all participants know that they may do the activity of their choice: walking, jogging, or running.

- If you have a PA system available, congratulate everyone on a job well done and reiterate the FFL message of the day!
- If you choose, give out participation certificates to commemorate the event.

Variations

Work with the local police department and host a FFL Fun Run in the community. Get donations from local community businesses for prizes, food, and water. Host it on an evening or weekend.

Celebration Activity 5: GYM (Get Yourself Moving) Club

Description

Start a GYM (Get Yourself Moving) club. Offer students access to the club before school, during recess, or after school depending on your schedule. Club activity examples could include a jump rope club (individual jump rope, double dutch, and long jump rope skills), sport skills club (basketball, volleyball, or soccer), circus arts club (stilts, juggling, flower sticks, diabolos, unicycles), dance club (line, folk, square, modern, hip-hop), and muscle maniacs club (organized games and activities to get students moving).

Following is a sample GYM club for rope jumping.

Purpose

To give students another opportunity to be active and to improve their individual jump rope skills

Planning

- Decide on the time when the club will be offered (mornings at 8:00 am to 8:30 am).

- Determine who is invited to participate (first through fifth grade).
- Identify the kind of GYM Club. The following example club focuses on individual jump rope skills. You can also use the blank certificate to create your own club.
- Decide where you will meet and on which days of the week (for instance, in the gym; Monday and Wednesday mornings are for fourth and fifth graders, Tuesday and Thursday are for second and third graders, and Friday is for first graders).
- Decide what equipment you will need (short jump ropes—enough for everyone).
- Decide what you will have them practice. Plan your session.

Equipment

- Individual jump ropes for everyone
- Signup sheets (created by you)
- Poster board schedule (created by you)
- Certificates of participation for everyone

 General → Celebrations

Blank certificate
CA5 GYM Club

Directions

- The week before you offer the club, have students sign up to participate. Let them know that this is like being in a class; that by signing up they are being responsible and you expect them to be there.

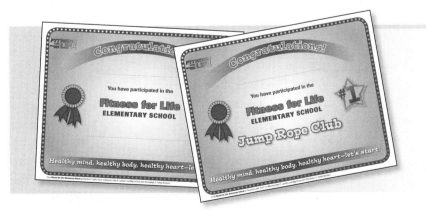

teacher tip • • •
Start with one club and see how you like it; then add another or just change the activity. You will have new students sign up with a change in activity. Give your students variety.

- Post a sign by the gym door indicating which class is on which day.
- Plan your activities.
- When students arrive, have them begin jumping rope immediately.
- When everyone has arrived, make a big deal of being in the GYM Jump Rope Club.
- Challenge them with a review of old tricks (basic jump pattern, ski jumper, rocker, criss-cross) and introduce new tricks (double under, reverse criss-cross, partner tricks).
- At the end of the club, hand out FFL Jump Rope Club participation certificates.

Variations

Depending on the size of your gym and the amount of equipment you have, you could have everyone every day for one week. If you really like the club idea, you could do it more often and expand it to other activities.

Celebration Activity 6: Fitness Trail

Description

Designate a trail outside on the playground or field for walking and jogging. Place a fitness exercise station or task card every 50 feet or so around the track. Students jog or walk the trail, and when they reach a fitness card they perform that exercise. Fitness cards show and explain how to do the exercise. Students are encouraged to choose their fitness challenge level—rookie, major league, or all-star. Depending on how you want to do this, you can have students participate during recess. This can be accomplished by the whole school, by grade levels, by individual classes, and or in physical education classes inside or out, depending on your facilities.

Purpose

To give students another opportunity to be active

Planning

- Designate your Fitness Trail.
- Create, print, and laminate Fitness Trail task cards. These cards should include the name of an exercise and brief instructions for performing it correctly. Possible examples could include jumping jacks, modified hurdler stretches, wall push-ups, or curl-ups.
- Decide how you will run this event. Will this be a recess activity, a physical education activity, a classroom activity, a grade level activity, or a TEAM Time activity (whole school together)? It could be a combination of all of these.
- Determine where you will meet and on which days of the week (for instance, in the gym; Monday and Wednesday mornings are for fourth and fifth graders, Tuesday and Thursday are for second and third graders, and Friday is for first graders).
- Choose the equipment you will need.
- Decide what you will have them practice. Plan your session.

Equipment

- Activity cards for each station
- Many stations can include activities that do not require equipment. However, the following equipment could be used at some of the stations: jump ropes, hula hoops, elastic bands.

Directions

- Place traffic cones at least 50 feet apart to designate your FFL Fitness Trail. Tape the task cards to the cones. (After your students learn how to use the trail, they will gladly help you set it up.)
- Introduce the FFL Fitness Trail to your students during physical education so they know what is expected and how to use the trail. Have them practice.
- Tell the classroom teachers about the FFL Fitness Trail and encourage them to use it throughout the day.

teacher tip • • •
Don't place the signs too close together. Add variety by changing the signs. Add your own ideas and equipment to the mix.

• Encourage your students to use it during their recess.

Variations

Start different students at different stations to get everyone participating. Ask teachers to do the stations with the students.

Celebration Activity 7: Pay to Play

Description

Students jog or walk around a designated area. After completing each lap they receive a Healthy Body Benefit Buck. When students have collected enough money they can purchase another activity to play by paying the banker (teacher). Cost of play is up to the teacher. Some activities cost more than others. A general rule of thumb is to charge five dollars to play for five minutes.

Purpose

To give students another opportunity to be active

Planning

• Designate the jogging or walking course.
• Make copies of the Healthy Body Benefit Bucks and laminate them.
• Decide which activities will be available to purchase and how much will they cost.
• Make a menu of their play choices and how much it costs for each.
• Make a list of the equipment you need.
• Decide how long they should stay at each play activity (five minutes should be plenty of time).

💿 **General → Celebrations**

CA7 Pay to Play

Equipment

• Dependent on the activity centers chosen
• Pay to Play Menu of activities
• Healthy Body Benefit Bucks

Directions

• Students walk, jog, or run around the perimeter of the activity area at a good pace.
• Each time students complete one lap, they receive one dollar from the banker (teacher).
• After students complete five laps, they can choose whether to keep moving or pay the banker to play another activity.
• The object of the activity is for students to participate in a variety of physical activities before the time is up. Each center usually costs between 5 and 10 dollars to participate.
• Students pay the banker each time they go to a new physical activity. Students can move aerobically and receive lots of money before spending it.
• Once they spend their money and play, they have to earn more by running again.

Possible Centers and Activities

• Short jump rope
• Long jump rope
• Hula hoop activities
• Pogo sticks
• Stilts

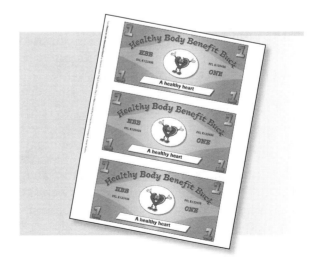

teacher tip • • •
Have a sale on activities to get more people involved. Have students help you decide the play activities and set the price.

- Basket shooting
- Playground games
- Playground equipment like swings or slides

Variations

Simply organized tag games could be used as well but would require more people.

Celebration Activity 8: Seasonal Events and Health Observances

During the school year there are many special health observances, including special months, weeks, and days devoted to promoting good fitness and health, as well as sound nutrition and physical activity. In the pages that follow, some of these special health observances are listed. Web sites for getting more information about these special events are provided. Details about these and other special events and national health observances can be found at www.healthfinder.gov.

Special signs are available for printing for some of the seasonal and health observances. All signs are saved together in one file.

 General → Celebrations

   CA8 Events

You can also print the blank signs provided on the DVD and customize them to create new signs for your own events and observances.

 General → General Signs

August

August is Children's Eye Health and Safety Month. For more information visit the Web site of Prevent Blindness America (www.prevent-blindness.org).

September

September is 5 to 9 a Day Month. This day refers to eating 5 to 9 fruits and vegetables every day—an important nutrition goal for children. The first Wellness Week features fruits and vegetables. Discussing the meaning of 5 to 9 a Day during September helps focus on the fruit and vegetable theme.

Conduct activities to encourage kids to eat a wide variety of fruits and vegetables, all six colors and white as well.

Three signs are available for posting during September of each year:

- September is 5 to 9 a Day Month.
- Eat 5 to 9 a day.
- Fruits and veggies help you play.

October

October is Child Health Month (National Child Health Day is during the first week). Walk to School Day/Week is during Child Health Month. Consider doing a Walking School Bus Activity on Walk Your Child to School Day (www.walk-toschool-usa.org). Walking School Bus refers to groups of parents, adults, and children walking to school together. For more information consult www.walkingschoolbus.org. Find out more about child health at www.mchb.hrsa.gov.

One sign is available for posting during October of each year:

- October is Child Health Month. Get active and eat well every day.

November

November is the Great American Health Challenge (to prevent and stop smoking). This event is sponsored by the American Cancer Society. For more information on this activity that prevents people from smoking and helps people stop smoking and using tobacco products, go to www.cancer.org/docroot/subsite/greatamericans/content/All_About_Smokeout.asp.

One sign is available for posting during November of each year:

- Be smart: Don't start!

December

National Hand Washing Awareness Week is in December. For more information go to www. henrythehand.com. The site contains download-able songs and movies about hand washing for good health.

January

The third full week in January is Healthy Weight Week. The Healthy Weight Network promotes special programs during this week. For more information, go to www.healthyweightnetwork. com.

February

February is American Heart Month. The American Heart Association promotes special programs during this month. For more information, go to www.americanheart.org.

March

March is National Nutrition Month. The American Dietetics Association promotes special nutrition activities during this month. Tie in **FFL: Elementary** nutrition activities to highlight this month. For more information, go to www.jimcolemanltd.com/nnm/ and www. eatright.org.

School Breakfast Week is also in March. The sponsor of school breakfast week is the School Nutrition Association. You can tie nutrition information from **FFL: Elementary** to the monthly theme. More information is available concerning menus, contests, and tools to promote healthy breakfasts at www.schoolnutrition.org.

Four signs are available to post during March:

- March is National Nutrition Month.
- School Breakfast Week is in March.
- Eat a healthy breakfast every day.
- Be wise: Eat well and exercise!

April

Turn Off (the TV) Week is in April. This week is dedicated to reducing the sedentary activity of TV watching and is sponsored by the Center for Screentime, a nonprofit organization for promoting healthier living. Information concerning this special week and other methods of reducing TV watching are available at www. screentime.org.

Two signs are available for posting during Turn Off (the TV) Week:

- Turn Off (the TV) Week is in April.
- Turn off the TV. Tune in to physical activity!

May

May is National Physical Fitness and Sports Month. It is sponsored by the President's Council on Physical Fitness and Sports. The council encourages youth to earn their Active Lifestyle Award at any time of the year but makes a special push for participation during May. You may want to encourage students to take part in the Active Lifestyle Program. They can enroll and keep records online. For more information go to www.presidentschallenge.org/the_challenge/ active_lifestyle.aspx. For general information about the President's Council, go to www. fitness.gov.

Two related signs are available for posting during May:

- May is National Physical Fitness and Sports Month.
- Play a sport, and get fit!

National Physical Education and Sport Week is also in May. This week is sponsored by the National Association for Sport and Physical Education (NASPE). NASPE provides information about activities that can be performed during the week, certificates of participation, and many other items to promote this week. For more information, go to www.aahperd.org/ naspe/advocacy/events/mayWeek/index.cfm.

Two related signs are available for posting during National Physical Education and Sport Week:

- National Physical Education and Sport Week is the first week in May.
- Celebrate physical education: Enjoy a sport.

May also features Project ACES (All Children Exercising Simultaneously), which was created by Len Saunders in 1989. On the first Wednesday of May of each year, Project ACES conducts an event to get youth throughout the world to be active at the same time. You may want to have all of the children in your school participate in Project ACES by doing a TEAM Time activity on ACES Day. For more information about Project ACES go to http://lensaunders.com/aces/aces.html.

One related sign is available for posting on ACES Day:

- Today is ACES Day: All Children Exercise Simultaneously.

June

The first week in June is National Family Recreation Week. This week is sponsored by the American Association for Leisure and Recreation Insurance. The association encourages family events such as a family hike or a picnic during this week. You might plan a family event at school such as a family walk during this week. More ideas for this week are available at www.aalr.org/nfrw.htm.

Two related signs are available for posting this week:

- National Family Recreation Week is the first week of June.
- Catch a fish, go for a hike, climb a hill, ride a bike.

teacher tip • • •
Web sites are available to help you learn more about many of the special events and observances described in this activity. Take a few minutes to explore the URLs provided to be sure that you have all the information you need to conduct the activities effectively.

EVENTS SIGNS

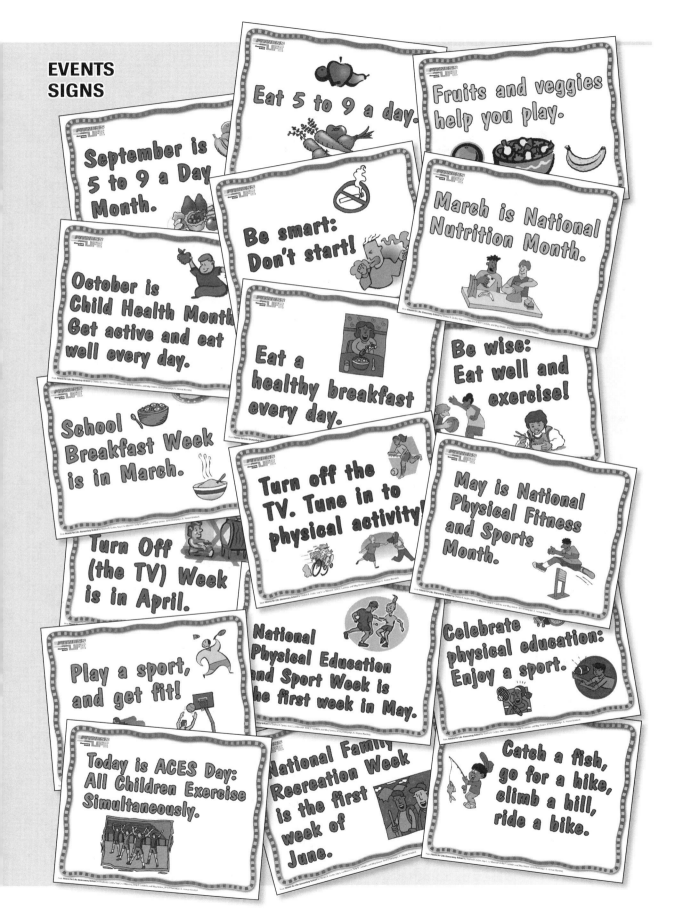

Eat 5 to 9 a day.

Fruits and veggies help you play.

September is 5 to 9 a Day Month.

Be smart: Don't start!

March is National Nutrition Month.

October is Child Health Month. Get active and eat well every day.

Eat a healthy breakfast every day.

Be wise: Eat well and exercise!

School Breakfast Week is in March.

Turn off the TV. Tune in to physical activity!

May is National Physical Fitness and Sports Month.

Turn Off (the TV) Week is in April.

Play a sport, and get fit!

National Physical Education and Sport Week is the first week in May.

Celebrate physical education: Enjoy a sport.

Today is ACES Day: All Children Exercise Simultaneously.

National Family Recreation Week is the first week of June.

Catch a fish, go for a hike, climb a hill, ride a bike.

Program Assessments

Fitness for Life: Elementary School is a schoolwide program designed to promote wellness, healthy eating, and regular physical activity. Properly conducted, it can be an effective part of a school's wellness program and help fulfill the wellness policy mandated by law. An approved wellness plan requires some form of program assessment. This section provides three assessment options: **FFL: Elementary** assessments, school health plan assessments, and school wellness plan assessments. If your school does not have a wellness policy or wellness plan, you will need to create one. The Action for Healthy Kids Web site (www.actionforhealthykids.org) provides a useful tool for developing wellness plans and policies. The booklet *Model Guidelines for Health and Wellness* is another tool to help you develop a wellness plan, and it is available on the DVD in this guide (see pages 16 and 74 for more about this tool).

FFL: Elementary Assessments

The DVD includes several tools to help you assess the effectiveness of **FFL: Elementary** Wellness Weeks. These tools are easy to use and can also be found on pages 95 to 103. Following is a step-by-step approach to assessment.

Step 1: Consider Assessment Tool Options

The tools available include assessments for the classroom teacher, the physical education teacher, students, the wellness coordinator, and

families. All of these tools are available in one folder on the DVD.

 General → Assessments

Classroom Teacher Program Assessment Tool

Physical Education Teacher Program Assessment Tool

Student Video Activity Ratings

Wellness Coordinator Program Assessment Tool

Family Wellness Week Assessment

Family Physical Activity and Nutrition Questionnaire

Analysis Form for Assessments

Classroom Teacher

This is a five-question tool that allows classroom teachers to assess **FFL: Elementary** Wellness Week programs. This tool is for classroom teachers to assess individual Wellness Weeks or all four Wellness Weeks as a whole. After the teachers have completed the forms, the wellness coordinator can tally the results and use them to improve future Wellness Weeks and to provide feedback to teachers and administration about the **FFL: Elementary** program. The Classroom Teacher Program Assessment Tool is available on page 95 and also on the DVD.

Physical Education Teacher

This is a five-question tool that allows physical education teachers to assess **FFL: Elementary** Wellness Week programs. This tool is for physical education teachers to assess individual Wellness

Weeks or all four Wellness Weeks as a whole. After the teachers have completed the forms, the wellness coordinator can use them to improve future Wellness Weeks and to provide feedback to teachers and administration about the **FFL: Elementary** program. The Physical Education Teacher Program Assessment Tool is available on page 96 and also on the DVD.

Students

This is a two-question tool that allows students to assess the video activities performed in the classroom. This tool is for students (either all students or a representative sample) to assess individual Wellness Weeks or all four Wellness Weeks as a whole. The information from this tool, together with the classroom teacher, physical education teacher, wellness coordinator, and family assessments, can be used to improve future Wellness Weeks and to provide feedback to teachers and administration about the **FFL: Elementary** program. The Student Video Activity Ratings is available on page 97 and also on the DVD.

Wellness Coordinator

This is a seven-question tool that allows wellness coordinators to assess **FFL: Elementary** Wellness Week programs. This tool is for the wellness coordinator to assess individual Wellness Weeks or all four Wellness Weeks as a whole. The information from this tool, together with the classroom teacher, physical education teacher, student, and family assessments, can be used to improve future Wellness Weeks and to provide feedback to teachers and administration about the **FFL: Elementary** program. The Wellness Coordinator Program Assessment Tool is available on page 98 and also on the DVD.

Family Members

This five-question tool allows family members to give their input about Wellness Week activities. You may distribute it to all families or selected groups of families to get feedback about Wellness Weeks. The information from this tool, together with the classroom teacher, physical education teacher, wellness coordinator, and student assessments, can be used to improve future Wellness Weeks and to provide feedback to the administration about the **FFL: Elementary**

program. The Family Wellness Week Assessment is available on page 99 and also on the DVD.

The Family Physical Activity and Nutrition Questionnaire is also available on pages 100 to 101 and the DVD to help family members assess the activity and nutrition behaviors of children. You may wish to distribute this questionnaire or put it on your school Web site for parents to use.

Step 2: Choose Appropriate Assessment Tools

You may choose to use different assessment tools for each Wellness Week. For example, you might ask classroom teachers to do an assessment for week 1, students to do an assessment for week 2, parents for week 3, and physical education teachers and wellness coordinator for week 4. As another option, you can use all assessments each Wellness Week. Much depends on the amount of time that can be devoted to assessment. Getting some information from all groups can help you and your school staff determine the effectiveness of Wellness Week programs and provide information to improve future Wellness Weeks. *Since federal laws require a wellness policy that includes assessment, the assessments described here can be part of the overall wellness plan assessment program.* You can do as many assessments each Wellness Week as time allows.

Step 3: Choose Distribution Methods

Once you have chosen the appropriate assessment tools to use, you need to decide how you want to distribute the assessment. For example, you may want to make paper copies or you may want to use e-mail. Sending the questionnaires to faculty, staff, and parents by e-mail is more cost effective than using paper. If not sent by e-mail, parent assessments may be distributed at Wellness Week celebration activities.

Step 4: Choose Groups to Sample

It might be a good idea to gather information from a sample of students from each grade and a sample of teachers in the school. If you gather a little bit of information following each of the four Wellness Weeks during the school year, you will have enough data to evaluate the program and make changes to improve Wellness Weeks for all of the school's stakeholders.

Step 5: Summarize Results

Use the analysis form to create a summary of responses. Have classroom teachers total student responses on the analysis form. You then can summarize the responses of all students for whom data were collected. You can also use the analysis form to summarize responses from classroom teachers who completed the Classroom Teacher Program Assessment Tool. Keep a folder for all assessment results. Provide your staff and students with some of the most important information and consider assessment results in planning for future Wellness Weeks.

You may also wish to share your assessment results with the authors of the **FFL: Elementary** program. They rely on feedback to make improvements in future editions of the program. Visit www.fitnessforlife.org and click on Feedback and Assessment to share information.

The Analysis Form for Assessments is available on pages 102 to 103 and also on the DVD.

Other Health and Wellness Assessments

The Centers for Disease Control and Prevention have developed an assessment tool for evaluating your school's total health program called the School Health Index. This comprehensive assessment tool is available at https://apps.nccd. cdc.gov/shi/default.aspx. You may want to consider using this index when making assessments at your school.

As noted earlier in this guide, every school that receives federal funding for school nutrition programs is required to have a wellness policy and a wellness plan. A school wellness assessment is required as part of a school wellness policy. In addition to the assessments of **FFL: Elementary** described in the previous section, you may want to do a more comprehensive evaluation of your school's wellness activities. Additional resources for assessment and evaluation of your coordinated school wellness plan (Wellness Policy Tool) are available from Action for Healthy Kids (www.actionforhealthykids. org/school-programs/our-programs/wellness-policy-tool/).

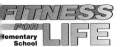

Classroom Teacher Program Assessment Tool

For each item below, check **one** box to indicate your satisfaction with that aspect of Wellness Week. This form may be used for each individual Wellness Week or cumulatively for all four Wellness Weeks. Write in the week number and names of the videos and activities used that week. Please turn this in to the wellness coordinator when completed.

Item to rate	Good	OK	Poor	N/A
1. Video activities for classroom breaks for Wellness Week ____				
Video activity: _____				
Instructional video (if used): _____				
2. Afternoon activities				
3. Teacher resources				
Lesson plans				
Ease of use				
Quality of the plans				
Classroom signs				
Worksheets				
Newsletters				
4. Schoolwide events				
Eat Well Wednesday (cafeteria) activities				
Get Fit Friday (TEAM Time) activities				
Other school celebrations: _____				
5. Wellness Week ____ overall satisfaction				

N/A = not applicable

Comments:

95

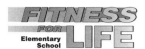

Physical Education Teacher Program Assessment Tool

For each item below, check **one** box to indicate your satisfaction with that aspect of Wellness Week. This form may be used for each individual Wellness Week or cumulatively for all four Wellness Weeks. Write in the week number and names of the videos and activities used that week. Please turn this in to the wellness coordinator when completed.

Item to rate	Good	OK	Poor	N/A
1. Video activities for Wellness Week ____				
Video activity: _____				
Instructional video: _____				
2. Lesson plans for Wellness Week ____				
Warm-Up Lesson Plan (week before Wellness Week)				
Lesson Plan 1				
Lesson Plan 2				
Lesson Plan 3				
3. Teacher resources				
Signs and cards				
Worksheets				
Newsletters				
4. Schoolwide events				
Eat Well Wednesday (cafeteria) activities				
Get Fit Friday (TEAM Time) activities				
Other school celebrations: _____				
5. Wellness Week ____ overall satisfaction				

N/A = not applicable

Comments:

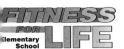

Student Video Activity Ratings

Read each question and think of an answer. Then circle the face that matches your answer. Please turn this in to your teacher when you are done.

1. Were the video activities fun?	☺	😐	☹
2. Would you like to do them again?	☺	😐	☹

Comments:

om **Fitness for Life: Elementary School** by Charles B. Corbin, Guy C. Le Masurier, Dolly D. Lambdin, and Meg Greiner, 2010 (Champaign, IL: Human Kinetics).

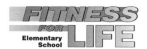

Wellness Coordinator Program Assessment Tool

For each item below, check **one** box to indicate your satisfaction with that aspect of Wellness Week. This form may be used for each individual Wellness Week or cumulatively for all four Wellness Weeks. Write in the week number.

Item to rate	Good	OK	Poor	N/A
1. Feedback from teachers about classroom activities				
2. Feedback from physical education teachers about activities				
3. Coordinator rating of schoolwide activities				
4. Resources				
Signs				
Eat Well Wednesday (cafeteria) activities				
Get Fit Friday (TEAM Time) activities				
Newsletters				
5. Schoolwide events				
Eat Well Wednesday (cafeteria) activities				
Get Fit Friday (TEAM Time) activities				
Other school celebrations: _____				
6. *Guide for Wellness Coordinators*				
7. Wellness Week _____ overall satisfaction				

N/A = not applicable

Note: Save the coordinator assessments in an assessment file. Share the results with the school principal and others involved in **Fitness for Life: Elementary School**. Solicit comments and use other assessment results to improve future Wellness Week activities.

Comments:

98

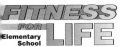

Family Wellness Week Assessment

Over the past week, your child has been involved in special Wellness Week activities. Please take a few minutes to answer the following questions. Check **one** box for each item. Please return the assessment to your child's teacher. This assessment will help provide improved wellness programs for your child.

Item to rate	Yes	No	N/A
1. Did you know about Wellness Week activities?			
2. Has your child made comments about special activities this past week (classroom exercise breaks or nutrition activities)?			
3. Has your child demonstrated physical activities or sung songs about exercise over the past week?			
4. Did your child bring home a Wellness Week newsletter or worksheet this past week?			
5. Did you participate in any Wellness Week activities at school or at home?			

N/A = not applicable

Comments:

99

From **Fitness for Life: Elementary School** by Charles B. Corbin, Guy C. Le Masurier, Dolly D. Lambdin, and Meg Greiner, 2010 (Champaign, IL: Human Kinetics).

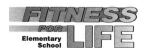

Family Physical Activity and Nutrition Questionnaire

Use this questionnaire to get ideas about your child's nutrition and physical activity habits. Check the box that represents the frequency for each item. This questionnaire is for your use only and does not need to be returned to school.

Nutrition

Does your child . . .

	Usually	Sometimes	Rarely
1. eat breakfast?			
2. avoid drinks high in sugar (for example, sweetened soft drinks)?			
3. avoid empty calories (for example, candy, donuts, cookies, chips, fries)?			
4. eat 5 or more veggies and fruits each day?			
5. avoid fast food?			
6. regularly eat whole grains and foods with protein (for example, milk products, meat, beans, nuts)?			
6. eat healthy lunches and dinners?			
7. eat with family members?			

Physical Activity

Does your child . . .

	Usually	Sometimes	Rarely
1. do 60 minutes of activity each day?			
2. do some vigorous activity each day?			
3. walk to school or stay active at home (for example, yard work or house work)?			
4. do exercise that builds muscles (for example, calisthenics, gymnastics, climbing apparatus)?			
5. do stretching exercises (for example, gymnastics, calisthenics)?			
6. watch TV or play computer games less than 2 hours each day?			
7. play outside?			

To rate your child's nutrition and physical activity habits, refer to the next page.

From **Fitness for Life: Elementary School** by Charles B. Corbin, Guy C. Le Masurier, Dolly D. Lambdin, and Meg Greiner, 2010 (Champaign, IL: Human Kinetics).

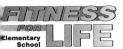

To rate your child's physical activity and nutrition habits, count the number of boxes you have checked in each of the three columns in both sections.

- If most of the checks are in the "Usually" column, congratulations! Your child is living a healthy lifestyle.
- If the majority of the checks are distributed between the "Usually" and "Sometimes" columns, your child should try to change some habits. Examine the questions that didn't get a "Usually," and make an effort to improve in those areas.
- If there are more than a few checks in the "Rarely" column and just a few in the "Usually" column, it's time to take action if you want your child to grow up fit, strong, and healthy. Carefully examine the areas that didn't get a "Usually," and make a plan to gradually change some habits, choosing a couple of areas to work on each month until you've worked on all the weak habits.

Rating	Answers to questionnaire
Healthy	You checked "Usually" for most items, with few or no checks for "Rarely."
Marginal	You most often checked "Usually" or "Sometimes."
Needs improvement	You checked "Rarely" more than a few times, with only a few checks for "Usually."

This questionnaire is meant to help parents and supervising adults get a general idea of the eating and exercise patterns of their children. For a more comprehensive analysis, consider using the Nutrition and Physical Activity Trackers at the MyPyramid Web site (www.mypyramidtracker.gov).

om **Fitness for Life: Elementary School** by Charles B. Corbin, Guy C. Le Masurier, Dolly D. Lambdin, and Meg Greiner, 2010 (Champaign, IL: Human Kinetics).

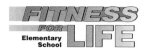

Analysis Form for Assessments

Use this form to collate responses to the Classroom Teacher Program Assessment Tool, the Family Wellness Week Assessment, and the Student Video Activity Ratings. Because a school typically has only one wellness coordinator and one or two physical education teachers, this form does not include the questionnaires completed by those staff members.

Classroom Teacher Assessment Tally Form

Place a tally mark in the appropriate column for each teacher answer. Count the tally marks in each column.

Wellness Week ____	Good	OK	Poor	N/A
1. Video activities for classroom breaks				
Video activity: _____				
Instructional video: _____				
2. Afternoon activities				
3. Teacher resources				
Lesson plans				
Ease of use				
Quality of the plans				
Classroom signs				
Worksheets				
Newsletters				
4. Schoolwide events				
Eat Well Wednesday (cafeteria) activities				
Get Fit Friday (TEAM Time) activities				
Other school celebrations: _____				
5. Wellness Week ____ overall satisfaction				

Family Wellness Week Assessment Tally Form

Place a tally mark in the appropriate column for each parent response. Count the tally marks in each column.

Item to rate	Yes	No	N/A
1. Did you know about Wellness Week activities?			
2. Has your child made comments about special activities this past week (classroom exercise breaks or nutrition activities)?			
3. Has your child demonstrated physical activities or sung songs about exercise over the past week?			
4. Did your child bring home a Wellness Week newsletter or worksheet this past week?			
5. Did you participate in any Wellness Week activities at school or at home?			

N/A = not applicable

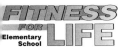

Student Assessment Tally Form

Place a tally mark in the appropriate column for each student answer. Count the tally marks in each column.

Item to rate	🙂	😐	🙁
Were the video activities fun?			
Would you like to do them again?			

om **Fitness for Life: Elementary School** by Charles B. Corbin, Guy C. Le Masurier, Dolly D. Lambdin, and Meg Greiner, 2010 (Champaign, IL: Human Kinetics).

APPENDIX C

Program Themes, Routines, and Messages

The **Fitness for Life: Elementary School** program uses various themes, video routines, and messages. This appendix includes tables that summarize the physical activity themes, nutrition themes, weekly video routines, and daily messages for all grades.

During each Wellness Week, the students in each grade perform a different routine during their morning activity break. Each grade does the same routine all five days of the week, but the routines provide new health and wellness messages every day. Each day is based on a general message,

such as "Be active every day," and the video hosts deliver three variations on that concept. The hosts deliver message variation 1 at the beginning of the video, students watch the routine and follow along, the hosts deliver message variation 2, students perform the routine again, and finally the hosts conclude with message variation 3.

The messages are also used in the classroom lesson plans and the physical education lesson plans, as well as in the signs, worksheets, newsletters, and other resources that accompany the program.

Wellness Week 1 Themes, Routines, and Messages

Grades K-2: Wellness Week 1

Activity theme: Moderate physical activity

Nutrition theme: Fruits and vegetables (fitness foods)

Routines: Kindergarten: Exercise on the Farm; Grade 1: Some More; Grade 2: Get Fit

Day and message	Variation 1	Variation 2	Variation 3
Day 1 Be active every day.	Move your muscles every day when you work and when you play.	Walking, playing, slow or fast—being active is a blast.	Move your body 60 minutes a day; that's an hour for fun and play. Be as active as you can be; play or walk with your family.
Day 2 Keep on trying!	The more you try, the better you get. We all can try, you bet, you bet.	It takes more than one try to get good. Try again—I knew you could.	Practice means trying again and again until you get better. So whether you hike, bike, or climb, practice helps you get better every time.
Day 3 Fitness foods	Fruits have colors of the rainbow and give you energy to help you grow.	Veggies have colors of the rainbow and give you energy to help you grow.	Rainbow-colored foods are good to eat. Red strawberries, green veggies, orange carrots, and blueberries are a special treat.
Day 4 Play safely.	Wear helmets, pads, sunscreen, and shoes. Playing safe is what we choose.	Helmets for heads and hats for sun; playing safe is much more fun.	Playing is much more fun when no one gets hurt. Equipment can help keep you safe, but safety starts with you. Use your ears to listen to instructions about playing safely, and use your eyes to spot danger during play.
Day 5 I can, you can, we all can.	I know we can do it; I'll tell you why. We can do it if we try, try, try!	I know we can do it; I'll tell you why. We can do it if we try, try, try!	The secret to success is trying. When you and your teammates try something together, anything is possible. Always give yourself a chance to be successful by trying.

Grades 3-5: Wellness Week 1

Activity theme: Moderate physical activity

Nutrition theme: Fruits and vegetables (eat 5 a day)

Routines: Grade 3: It's Our Plan; Grade 4: Robot; Grade 5: Hip Hop 5

Day and message	Variation 1	Variation 2	Variation 3
Day 1 60 minutes every day	Whatever you love to play, get 60 minutes every day. Wherever you love to play, get 60 minutes every day.	Whatever you love to play, get 60 minutes every day. Wherever you love to play, get 60 minutes every day.	Sixty minutes of physical activity every day is fun. Sixty minutes of physical activity every day makes you feel good. Sixty minutes of physical activity every day helps you build strong bones and muscles. Sixty minutes of physical activity every day means playing with friends and having a good time.
Day 2 The more you practice, the better you get.	Practice your technique; get better every week. Using skills when you play can be the best feelings of your day.	Practice your technique; get better every week. Practice skills in the sun; make movement way more fun.	Practicing and learning skills make physical activity more fun because you become a more successful mover when you're done. Practicing movements also exercises your body and your mind. That's a great workout that is hard to find!
Day 3 Eat 5 a day.	Eat five portions of fruits and vegetables each day. Fruits and veggies are what you need for growing tall and running speed. Fruits and veggies are made from the sun—nature's energy supply that helps us run.	Fruits and veggies are all-star snacks; ask for them in your lunch pack. Fruits and veggies are made from the sun—nature's energy supply that helps us run.	Eat many different colored fruits and veggies each day to make sure your growing body gets the vitamins and energy you need. Start by making a healthy fruit and veggie choice at the cafeteria. See if you can eat all the colors of the rainbow in fruits and veggies in one day.
Day 4 Start with safety.	If you want to play every day, take safety measures before you play. Clip on your helmet, tie up your shoes—play in control to avoid a bruise.	If you're playing in the sun, you need sunblock. Spread it on, and you're ready to rock.	Before you get out to play, make sure you have the right equipment and that you are wearing it properly. This can be as simple as tying up your shoes to protect your feet and ankles. It's also important to control your body when you are playing with others to prevent anyone from getting hurt. It's never fun when play ends with an injury. Start with safety, finish with fun!
Day 5 Fun for me, fun for you, fun for all.	Encouraging others during play is a great way to make someone's day. Encouraging others during play is a great plan for making friends today!	Don't spoil an awesome day—avoid mean words when you play. Don't spoil an awesome day—avoid mean looks when you play!	Encouraging others is a great way to make physical activity more fun and is a great way to make friends. We all like to be encouraged by others and feel like part of the group. People have a better time playing when put-downs are not around.

Grade 6: Wellness Week 1

Activity theme: Moderate physical activity

Nutrition theme: Fruits and vegetables (you are what you eat)

Routine: Hip Hop 6

Day and message	Variation 1	Variation 2	Variation 3
Day 1 There are lots of fun physical activities.	Whatever your style, whatever you play, choose to be active 60 minutes a day.	Whatever your style, whatever you play, choose to be active 60 minutes a day.	Sixty minutes of physical activity every day is fun. Sixty minutes of physical activity every day makes you feel good. Sixty minutes of physical activity every day helps you build strong bones and muscles. Sixty minutes of physical activity every day means playing with friends and having a good time.
Day 2 Practice builds skills.	Practice builds your physical skills. It's way more fun to move with skill, to move with flow, and get the feel. But you've got to practice—that's the deal!	Skills are learned by giving good tries. Improve your skills with practice—that's wise!	All practice is not equal. Good practice means doing something the right way. The more times you try something, doing it the right way, the better you get.
Day 3 You are what you eat.	There's a color in the pyramid for each food you eat, and there are steps up the side to help you move your feet.	Fruits and veggies with color locked in have vitamins, minerals, and energy to help our bodies win!	In addition to fruits (red) and veggies (green), there is an orange band for grains, a blue band for milk, a purple band for meat and beans, and a yellow band for oils.
Day 4 Safety is key for staying healthy.	Safety is key for staying healthy. It's hard to be helpful and hard to have fun if you're injured or sick and unable to run!	You can't help your team or play with your friends if you have to wait for injuries to mend!	Staying healthy takes more than good luck. You have to prepare yourself for physical activity by wearing the right equipment, warming up before you do the activity, and maintaining control of your body during the activity. You can't help your team from the bench or the sidelines. Stay safe, and stay in the game.
Day 5 I can!	Self-confidence is important; we know that's true. Self-confidence means believing in what you can do!	Don't get down on yourself—give yourself cred. Keep it positive with a pep talk in your head!	The way we think about ourselves and our abilities has an impact on our lives and our health. Keep the story in your head positive, and believe in yourself. You can do it. A great philosopher once said, "As you think, so shall you be." Setting small goals and working to meet them help you build confidence one step at a time. When you reach the first small goal, you can set another.

Wellness Week 2 Themes, Routines, and Messages

Grades K-2: Wellness Week 2

Activity theme: Vigorous physical activity (vigorous aerobics, sports, and recreation)

Nutrition theme: Grains and foods with fat

Routines: Kindergarten: Frank and Franny Fitness; Grade 1: I Can; Grade 2: La Raspa

Day and message	Variation 1	Variation 2	Variation 3
Day 1 Get your body moving!	Whether you live in the city or on a farm, moving your body is a lucky charm.	All little kids love to move around: rolling, running, jumping, and making fun sounds.	When you're very active, you feel alert and alive. If it makes your heart beat faster, give a high five! If it makes you breathe hard and sweat, it helps your brain and body work well—you bet!
Day 2 Get better with practice.	Do it once, then do it twice; practice, practice is good advice.	The more you practice, the better you play; practice, practice every day.	Practice means trying again and again until you are good. Try it, try it—I knew you could.
Day 3 Foods with fats	Some foods with fats are good; some fats are bad. What kind of fats has your body had?	Some foods with fats are good; some fats are bad. What kind of fats has your body had?	Your body needs fat for energy, protection, and warmth. Fats are found in many foods like muffins, bacon, cheese, and ice cream. Eating too much fatty food is not good for your body.
Day 4 Exercise your heart.	Exercising your heart really pays—your heart will thank you in so many ways!	Moving your body gets your heart thump, thump, thumping. Your cardio pump just keeps on pumping!	Playing hard and being active are a good start; it gets your blood pumping and builds a strong heart. Making your heart beat fast helps your body last.
Day 5 Never, ever give up!	Never give up, say it out loud; trying hard will make you proud.	Do your best, try hard, never quit; being active will get you fit.	That means keep going even if it's hard, whether it's inside or in the yard. Keep on going to get fit—never give up, never quit.

Grades 3-5: Wellness Week 2

Activity theme: Vigorous physical activity (vigorous aerobics, sports, and recreation)

Nutrition theme: Grains and empty calories

Routines: Grade 3: Go Aerobics Go; Grade 4: Latin Aerobics; Grade 5: Tinikling

Day and message	Variation 1	Variation 2	Variation 3
Day 1 Play for a good day.	Exercising on your own or playing sports with teams makes life more fun and fills our dreams. Dance for fun or dance for training; it will brighten your day even if it's raining!	Try lots of activities and get out and play. Find movement you love and do it every day. Your days will be brighter and your sleep will be sound; you'll get up the next day ready to move around!	Vigorous sports and recreation add joy and meaning to our lives. Playing allows us to use our imagination and express our creativity while we build fitness, make friends, and live a healthy life.
Day 2 Build skills, have more fun.	You'll have fun when you build fitness skills. Run, balance, spin, or swing; use these skills for many things. Learning ballet, soccer, or judo, or riding a bike all require skills that are alike!	Catch, stretch, bend, or aim. Many activities use skills that are the same.	Sports and recreational activities require many skills. But many different activities require the same types of skills. When a skill can be used in many different activities, we say that skill transfers.
Day 3 Avoid empty calories.	Avoid foods with empty calories. Just because there are calories doesn't make it good food. Cookies and donuts don't qualify, dude!	Salt, sugar, and fat-filled snacks and sweets: We don't eat them all the time; that's why they're called treats!	Candy bars, potato chips, and soda are products that taste good but don't have any vitamins. We say these products have empty calories because they have energy but no vitamins and other good nutrients. Find healthy snacks that have calories that are good for you. Veggies and fruits are good choices!
Day 4 Aerobic activity every day.	*Teacher:* Get some aerobic activity every day. Who's got heart? *Kids:* We've got heart! *Teacher:* Who's got heart? *Kids:* We've got heart! *Teacher:* Get going, get going from the very start!	Heart be pumping; heart be strong. Find your pulse; don't take too long. Feel your heart pumping, feel your heart thumping; get ready for the next song. Not too high, not too low; in our target zone we can go, go, go.	Activities that challenge your heart and lungs are called aerobic activities. If you build your aerobic fitness by challenging your heart and lungs, you will build a stronger heart muscle and lungs that can deliver oxygen to your blood more effectively. By checking your heart rate during exercise and play, you can find out if you are challenging your heart at the right level. That's called working in the target zone.
Day 5 Show respect.	When you play sports, it's like a dream, but you can't do it without another team. Treat other kids like you want them treating you; respecting others begins with you!	A team that gives you a challenge makes the game fun; make sure you give them a cheer when the game is done!	Being a good sport means more than just following the rules. It means respecting teammates and opponents through encouragement and kindness. Being a good sport also means involving others in physical activity even when they may not be the best players. It's always better to make people feel welcome in physical activity rather than exclude them for the sake of a game. Remember, it's just a game.

Grade 6: Wellness Week 2

Activity theme: Vigorous physical activity (vigorous aerobics, sports, and recreation)

Nutrition theme: Grains and high-calorie foods

Routine: Salsaerobics

Day and message	Variation 1	Variation 2	Variation 3
Day 1 Active all day	It's important to stay active every day. Moving in the morning, moving at lunch, moving after school with a healthy bunch. Get your friends moving and your family, too—movement gets them healthy, and they'll want to thank you!	Active in the classroom, active in PE, active with my family is the way to be.	You need at least an hour of activity each day. Two hours a day is even better. Finding ways to be active with your friends and family at home and at school is fun and good for your health.
Day 2 Start with the basics.	Many skills are required to play a game and succeed; spend time learning the basics before you proceed!	Dance steps, catching, or playing the right strings—practice the basics before the hard things!	Learn the basic skills with regular practice. You can refine your skills by practicing more complex moves. Skipping over the basics may limit how much you can improve in the future.
Day 3 High-calorie foods	If you want to know how much energy is in your food, learn about calories from fat, carbohydrate, and protein, dude!	Compared to carbs and protein, fat calories are double. You can see why eating fatty foods can get you in trouble!	Energy in foods is measured by how many calories they contain. Carbohydrate, such as in fruits and veggies, contains fewer than half of the calories found in fat, such as in butter. Extra calories in foods that are not used in being physically active are stored in the body as fat.
Day 4 Heartbeats for health	Your heart is like any other muscle; you know it's growing bigger when you make it hustle. It's good to get it pumping hard and fast; when you get it in the zone, how long can you last?	Your target zone is where your heart needs to beat if you want fitness and like feeling sweet! Getting in the zone strengthens your heart, so get in the zone from the very start.	You can tell when an activity is making your heart beat faster by counting your pulse at your wrist or on the side of your neck. Each pulse that you feel represents one beat of your heart.
Day 5 Self-respect	By honoring yourself and showing some pride, you give your body a healthy ride. Eat right, move often, and get your rest. Now you're up for any test.	Honor your body, show it you care. Give it exercise, an apple, or a pear. You have to take care of your body and make it number one to do your best work and have some fun.	Self-respect is about taking care of yourself. Respect your body and your mind by exercising and eating healthy foods. You can't be your best or help others if you don't take care of yourself first.

Wellness Week 3 Themes, Routines, and Messages

Grades K-2: Wellness Week 3

Activity theme: Muscle fitness and flexibility exercises

Nutrition theme: Foods for strong bones and muscles

Routines: Kindergarten: We Get Fit; Grade 1: CYIM Fit; Grade 2: Wave It

Day and message	Variation 1	Variation 2	Variation 3
Day 1 Get your muscles ready.	You need to get your muscles warm before you play or perform. Start moving slowly, then move fast—now your muscles are ready to last.	You need to get your muscles warm before you play or perform. Start moving slowly, then move fast—now your muscles are ready to last.	Warm up before you exercise because it will help your muscles stretch farther. Warm muscles allow you to jump higher, reach farther, and run faster.
Day 2 Move your body.	You have many body parts to move. Move with the music; get in the groove.	To move to the music, you need quick feet; keep your body moving to the beat.	Singing and moving with friends are fun. You'll move all of your body before you're done.
Day 3 Food for strong bones and muscles	Strong bones, strong muscles, strong teeth—yes, please! Let's drink milk and eat beans and a little cheese.	Eggs and fish and vegetable greens build muscles and bones like you've never seen.	Our muscles get protein from beans, meat, milk, cheese, and eggs. Our bones get calcium from milk, cheese, and green leafy vegetables. Eat some of these foods every day to grow strong and play.
Day 4 You have only one body; make it fit!	One rule of fitness you need to know: challenging your muscles makes them grow.	*Overload* means doing more than you usually do. It's a basic rule of fitness that applies to me and you.	Take care of your body and exercise a lot; it's the only one you've got. Be a responsible body owner; take good care of your one and only body.
Day 5 If it is to be, it's up to me.	Trying hard gets things done; trying hard makes me number one.	It may be hard the first time I try, but with a few more tries, I can reach the sky. The choice is mine; it's up to me. I'll try real hard—watch and see.	If I think I can, I can. If I think I can't, I can't. Whatever I think is right. I need to believe with all my might. You are in charge of how hard you will try, how you feel, and how you treat others.

Grades 3-5: Wellness Week 3

Activity theme: Muscle fitness and flexibility exercises

Nutrition theme: Protein power

Routines: Grade 3: Tic Tac Toe 3; Grade 4: Tic Tac Toe 4; Grade 5: Tic Tac Toe 5

Day and message	Variation 1	Variation 2	Variation 3
Day 1 Take care of your muscles.	Take care of your muscles. Always warm up before you play. Stretch your muscles to make them longer. Build your muscles to make them stronger.	Cool down and reduce your speed; cooling down your body is what you need. Your muscles were warm, and you had fun. It's time to cool down before you're done.	You should always prepare your body for physical activity by warming up your muscles with some light jogging or exercises. Warm muscles are more flexible, allowing you to stretch them farther. Long, strong muscles help you in all types of activities. When you have finished your activity, move at half speed to gradually let your muscles cool down.
Day 2 Practice for fitness.	Stretching takes practice and skillful technique. Practice your stretching at least three times a week! How you stretch is important, too; practice proper stretching to make it work for you!	Building muscles requires skill and technique; strengthen your muscles three times per week!	The Physical Activity Pyramid for Kids shows that flexibility and muscle fitness should be done three times a week. Just as you need to practice skills to improve, you need to perform stretching and strengthening exercises regularly to become more flexible and stronger.
Day 3 Protein power	Become lean, mean, moving machines! Beans, nuts, meat, and milk are foods with protein.	Protein builds cells in muscles and brains; eat your protein foods and make big gains!	Protein is needed to build and maintain cells in your muscles and your brain. You can get protein if you wish from eating peanut butter and fish!
Day 4 Be specific; look terrific.	To get strength, flexibility, or speed, be specific when you train to get what you need!	Stretch a little bit farther, lift a little bit more; to build fitness, do more than before!	Two principles of exercise are overload and specificity. Overload means to build fitness, do a little more than normal. Specificity means to build a specific part of fitness, train for that part of fitness. If you want to have stronger legs, you have to do muscle exercises with your legs, and gradually challenge them to do more than before. To build longer muscles, you must stretch them.
Day 5 Don't be a character—have character.	Consider others when you play; not everything can go your way. We all make mistakes, and accidents happen; encourage other people with hands a-clapping!	Strength means more than lifting weights. Strength of character counts with classmates. Following rules and sharing the ball demonstrate honesty and teamwork to all.	It's not enough to just play by the rules. To demonstrate a strong character, you need to follow the rules, support others in good and bad times, and be a good sport whether you win or lose. Making a call that goes against your team, helping an opponent up when they've fallen, and encouraging a teammate who has made a bad play are all examples of someone who has a strong character. Weak and cowardly characters look out for themselves, hog the ball, and try to win at all costs.

Grade 6: Wellness Week 3

Activity theme: Muscle fitness and flexibility exercises

Nutrition theme: Protein is important

Routine: Tic Tac Toe 6

Day and message	Variation 1	Variation 2	Variation 3
Day 1 There is no "I" in "team".	T-E-A-M, that's how you spell. There is no "I" included if we are going to do well.	To do well, be a good team member. "T-E-A-M," not "I," is important to remember.	Finding others to join you in activity not only can make it fun but also can help you to become and stay more active. Friends can encourage each other. Team members encourage each other.
Day 2 Feedback to improve	We all need feedback to improve. Feedback means listening carefully to what experts say. Using feedback and listening will help you when you play.	Feedback can help you correct a mistake. Listen to your teacher or coach—it's a piece of cake.	Watching your own performance in a mirror or watching a video of your own performance can give you feedback to help you improve.
Day 3 Protein is important.	Protein is important at every meal—it provides the building blocks for the muscles you feel. Protein in the morning from hot cereal keeps you energized and feeling full.	Protein is important at every meal—it provides the building blocks for the muscles you feel. Protein in the morning from hot cereal keeps you energized and feeling full.	Amino acids are the building blocks for muscle proteins, brain cell proteins, and millions of other proteins in your body. Your body needs protein to create a healthy, strong you!
Day 4 You get what you train for.	You get what you train for. The specificity principle is a basic rule—learn about it. It means that if you do a specific exercise, you get a specific benefit.	To get flexibility, you must stretch, you know. Do muscle fitness exercise, and watch your muscles grow.	Moderate activity builds health in general. Vigorous activity builds the heart and blood vessels. Stretching builds flexibility, and overloading the muscles builds muscle fitness. Each specific type of activity has a specific benefit.
Day 5 Rules rule!	Rules are essential for playing a game. Without any rules, games would be lame. It's not enough to wait for the referee. I will follow the rules when no one's looking but me.	"Cheaters never win" is what some people say. Don't be called a cheater—be careful how you play.	Sometimes you can get by without following the rules. But following the rules, even when you can get away with breaking them, is a true test of character and being a good sport. Don't get labeled as a cheat—play hard and fair when you compete.

Wellness Week 4 Themes, Routines, and Messages

Grades K-2: Wellness Week 4

Activity theme: Integration (energy balance)

Nutrition theme: Healthy foods help us move

Routines: Kindergarten: Shake It; Grade 1: Stomp and Balance; Grade 2: It's the One

Day and message	Variation 1	Variation 2	Variation 3
Day 1 Get off your seat and move your feet.	Your brain gets working when you get on your feet; moving your body is a special treat.	Too much sitting makes you a couch potato; get up and move like a swirling tornado.	When you move around, you need your many senses like sight, sound, balance, and touch. Watching TV uses only sight and sound. Get out, get moving, and have some fun—you do your brain good when you get out and run.
Day 2 Play lots, learn lots.	When you play lots of games with family and friends, learning new skills will never end.	The more activities that you do, the more you'll learn—yes, that means you!	Trying lots of different physical activities helps us build many skills and meet many different people. The more you try, the more you'll know; the more you try, your friends will grow.
Day 3 Healthy food helps us move.	Did you know that the food we eat gives us energy to move our feet?	Eat healthy food for breakfast, lunch, and dinner. Eating healthy food can make us winners.	The food we eat gives us energy to ride our bikes, dance, and play hide and seek. Healthy food like fruits and vegetables gives us the energy we need and gives us vitamins to grow healthy.
Day 4 Be water wise.	Your body loses water when you sweat. Drinking lots of water is the best plan yet.	Sweating cools your body when you start to get hot. Take breaks and drink water if you want to play a lot.	Your body needs water to keep your insides cool; taking lots of drinks when playing is a pretty good rule.
Day 5 Plan to get better.	If you want to get better, you need a plan; write down what you want to do, and say, "I can."	If you want to do something better than before, make a plan to practice more and more.	If you want to do something better, writing a plan is the first step. Maybe your plan is to practice, or maybe it's to try something new. Whatever your plan is, it can only start with you.

Grades 3-5: Wellness Week 4

Activity theme: Integration (energy balance)

Nutrition theme: Balance energy in (food) with energy out (exercise)

Routines: Grade 3: Jumpnastics; Grade 4: Keep on Clapping; Grade 5: Fit Funk

Day and message	Variation 1	Variation 2	Variation 3
Day 1 Brain and body exercise	Learn a new movement, start to train; it's good for your heart and good for your brain!	Use your imagination, and your creativity will flow; play for pure enjoyment, and your brain will grow!	Physical activity engages the body and mind. Physical activity that requires creativity, imagination, and the use of our senses develops the brain and our fitness. Build physical and brain fitness while having lots of fun!
Day 2 Combine skills just for the fun of it.	Combine skills just for the fun of it. We can catch, we can hop, we can run, we can stop. One at a time these skills are tame; put the skills together for a wicked game!	Leap left, pass right, run for fun, jump for height. One at a time these skills are tame; put the skills together for a wicked game!	Performing one skill at a time may be easy. Try putting several skills together in a sequence, and it is much harder. Many activities require several skills. Dancing is an activity that requires choreographers to put several skills together to form a dance. Creating dances is fun and involves a lot of skill.
Day 3 Balance energy in (food) with energy out (exercise).	Balance the amount of food or energy you take in with the amount of exercise or energy you put out. Energy "in" is how much you eat. Energy "out" is how much you move. Balance the two and what you find is a healthy body and a healthy mind!	Keeping a healthy weight requires exercise. Also limit fatty foods like cookies and french fries.	Energy balance means balancing how many calories you get from food and drinks with the calories that you burn moving each day. Movement requires energy, and the more you move, the more energy you burn.
Day 4 Water, water, before I get hotter!	If you lose lots of water from sweating really hard, your body won't be able to keep running around the yard!	You won't be able to play your best if you don't drink water at every rest!	If you lose too much water from sweating, it's called dehydration. Dehydration prevents you from playing your best and can lead to muscle cramps. It's important to take regular water breaks when you're playing for a long time.
Day 5 Personal fitness starts with you.	Fitness, fitness! What kind do you want? Fitness, fitness! What kind do you need? Figure this out before you proceed!	Do you have good fitness? How would you know? Fitness assessments will tell you if you're good to go!	Fitness assessments help us determine whether we have a healthy level of fitness. They can also tell us if we have enough fitness for our favorite activities. It is important to decide what types of fitness you need for your favorite activities so that you can assess those that are most important to you. Once you know your fitness level, you can set goals for improving your fitness.

Grade 6: Wellness Week 4

Activity theme: Integration (energy balance)
Nutrition theme: Balance calories
Routine: Harvest Time

Day and message	Variation 1	Variation 2	Variation 3
Day 1 Build a healthy body; build a healthy mind.	It's good for the body; it's good for the mind—physical activity is one of a kind!	Using all your senses to run, dance, or throw builds new brain cells and helps muscles grow!	Physical activity is so important because it challenges the body and the mind. Physical activity requires you to use skills and senses to complete complicated tasks. Oh, yeah, it's also fun, if anybody asks.
Day 2 One step at a time	Learn physical skills one at a time. Learn the fundamentals; learn the basics, please. You'll thank me later when you're moving with ease!	Sports and dance are always more fun if you've learned the basics one by one. Don't pressure yourself to learn too fast; physical activity is fun, and we want it to last!	Learning something new takes time. Practicing one part of a new activity at a time and then putting the parts together can help you learn faster and better.
Day 3 Balance calories.	A calorie is a unit of energy; we can measure calories in food. Calories provide energy for physical activity, dude!	A high-calorie food or high-calorie drink adds more calories to your body than you might think. If you want to stay healthy and maintain your weight, you might not want to put a donut on your plate.	A soft drink with sugar has 150 calories. Doing 30 minutes of moderate activity expends about 150 calories for most people.
Day 4 Hit the water.	Hydration's a fancy word for taking a drink. It's more important for health than you might think!	Hydration's a fancy word for taking a drink. It's more important for sports performance than you might think!	Water is important for many body functions. Performing your best, looking your best, and feeling your best are all dependent on your hydration level. Got water?
Day 5 SMART goals	SMART goals are specific; SMART goals you can measure. Choose SMART goals for activity, and that will give you pleasure.	SMART goals are realistic and can be completed on time. Set SMART goals for activity, and watch your fitness climb.	S equals specific, M equals measurable, A equals attainable, R equals reasonable, and T stands for timely. Choose activity goals that you can achieve, that are reasonable, and that are good for you at this time!

APPENDIX D

NASPE Standards

Part III of this guide briefly discusses and lists the six NASPE standards for physical education. This appendix provides more detail about the standards and the specific performance outcomes used to develop the **Fitness for Life: Elementary School** program.

Each standard has descriptive paragraphs that outline student expectations and lists of sample performance outcomes for grades K-2, 3-5, 6-8, and 9-12. **FFL: Elementary** uses many of the sample performance outcomes. Additional performance outcomes were developed based on descriptions of student expectations for each grade group. Since **FFL: Elementary** is intended for grades K-6, standards for grade 6 were extracted from the grade 6-8 materials.

Following are the six general NASPE standards and the specific performance outcomes used in developing **FFL: Elementary**. The letters used in the lesson plan books correspond to the number of the general standard and letter of the performance outcomes.

The NASPE standards are reprinted from *Moving Into the Future: National Standards for Physical Education,* 2nd ed., 2004 (Reston, VA: National Association for Sport and Physical Education), 11.

Grades K-2

NASPE standards are grouped by the following grade levels: K-2, 3-5, 6-8, and 9-12. NASPE standards and performance outcomes used in creating the **FFL: Elementary** program for the K-2 grade levels are presented here.

Standard 1: Motor Skills and Movement Patterns

Children are active and enjoy learning and mastering new skills. Children achieve mature forms of movement patterns, including more mature patterns using various body parts.

Performance outcomes:

- A: Performs simple dance steps.
- B: Demonstrates clear contrast between fast and slow movements—keeping tempo.
- C: Demonstrates a smooth transition between locomotor skills in time to music.
- D: Discovers how to balance on different body parts.
- E: Performs more mature movement patterns using various body parts.
- F: Enjoys learning new activities and skills.

Standard 2: Movement Concepts, Principles, Strategies, and Tactics Applied to Learning and Performance

Children mature in cognitive abilities associated with movement. They learn to apply concepts to movements and to identify correct form in movement performances.

Performance outcomes:

- A: Identifies body planes (front, back, side).
- B: Identifies various body parts (knee, foot, arm, palm).

- C: States short-term effects of physical activity on heart and lungs.
- D: Explains that appropriate practice improves performance.
- E: Uses knowledge in movement situations.

Standard 3: Participates Regularly in Physical Activity

Children participate for pleasure and have fun while being active. They perform locomotor and nonlocomotor activities and use them during free time. They recognize the temporary and lasting effects of activity on the body and choose to perform activities that benefit health.
Performance outcomes:

- A: Engages in moderate to vigorous physical activity on an intermittent basis.
- B: Engages in a variety of locomotor activities (hopping, walking, jumping).
- C: Has fun while being active.
- D: Learns locomotor and nonlocomotor activities and uses them in free time.
- E: Knows several health benefits of physical activity.

Standard 4: Achieves and Maintains Health-Enhancing Physical Fitness

Children engage in activities that enhance health-related fitness and enjoy them. They recognize factors associated with moderate to vigorous activity (e.g., sweating, fast heart rate, heavy breathing). Students have basic knowledge about and understand the five parts of health-related fitness.
Performance outcomes:

- A: Demonstrates sufficient muscular strength to be able to bear body weight.
- B: Engages in a series of locomotor activities (e.g., timed segments of hopping, walking, and so on) without easily tiring.
- C: Recognizes physical responses to activity associated with fitness.
- D: Participates in a variety of games that increase breathing and heart rate.

- E: Sustains activity for increasingly longer periods of time while participating in various activities in physical education.
- F: Recognizes that health-related physical fitness consists of several different parts.

Standard 5: Exhibits Responsible Personal and Social Behavior and Respect for Others in Activity

Children discover the joy of playing with friends makes activities fun. They know safe practices and know how to apply rules. They use successful interpersonal communication during group activity. They appreciate cooperation in learning skills and cooperate, share, and work together to solve problems or meet a challenge.
Performance outcomes:

- A: Practices specific skills as assigned until the teacher signals the end of practice.
- B: Follows directions given to the class for an all-class activity.
- C: Shows compassion for others by helping them.
- D: Works in diverse group settings without interfering with others.
- E: Enjoys participating alone and in groups while exploring movement tasks.
- F: Accepts all playmates without regard to personal differences (e.g., ethnicity, gender, disability).
- G: Displays consideration of others while participating.
- H: Demonstrates the elements of socially acceptable conflict resolution during class activity.
- I: Shares and works well with other children in activity settings.

Standard 6: Values Physical Activity for Health, Enjoyment, Challenge, Self-Expression, and Social Interaction

Children are active and enjoy participating. They meet challenges of new movements and skills. They feel joy when they achieve competence and begin to function as a member of a group and use cooperation in activity.

Performance outcomes:

- A: Exhibits both verbal and nonverbal indicators of enjoyment.
- B: Willingly tries new movements and skills.
- C: Continues to participate when not successful on the first try.
- D: Identifies several activities that are enjoyable.
- E: Expresses personal feelings on progress while learning a new skill.
- F: Enjoys activity involvement and achieving motor skills.
- G: Functions well with other children in group activities.

Grades 3-6

NASPE standards are grouped by the following grade levels: K-2, 3-5, 6-8, and 9-12. The performance outcomes used in creating the **FFL: Elementary** program for grades 3-5 are listed below and are based on the grades 3-5 NASPE standards. The grade 6 performance outcomes are based on selected standards appropriate for grade 6 from the grades 6-8 NASPE standards. The standards and performance outcomes for grades 3-6 are listed here.

Standard 1: Motor Skills and Movement Patterns

Grades 3-6: Older children develop more mature fundamental motor skills for pleasurable movement experiences. They demonstrate locomotor, nonlocomotor, and manipulative skills and use these skills in a variety of environments and in various combinations.

Performance outcomes:

- A: Performs basic dance steps (e.g., tinikling).
- B: Demonstrates correct pattern for dance steps (e.g., polka).
- C: Uses skills in various combinations.
- D: Demonstrates advanced (mature) movement patterns.
- E: Demonstrates tactics (grade 6).
- F: Performs a variety of dances (grade 6).

Standard 2: Movement Concepts, Principles, Strategies, and Tactics Applied to Learning and Performance

Grades 3-5: Older children comprehend more complex concepts and principles and apply them in activity. They use feedback to correct their performances and can transfer concepts and principles from one activity for use in another.

Grade 6: Children exhibit complex discipline-specific knowledge; can apply principles related to practice and conditioning in activity; and can apply movement concepts, principles, and strategies. They can correct personal errors and describe principles of training that improve fitness.

Performance outcomes:

- A: Describes how heart rate is used to monitor exercise intensity.
- B: Explains the necessity of transferring weight from the back leg to the front leg during any action that propels an object forward.
- C: Explains how appropriate practice improves performance.
- D: Identifies physical and psychological benefits that result from long-term participation in physical activity.
- E: Can correct errors when given feedback (grade 6).
- F: Applies movement concepts, principles, and strategies (grade 6).
- G: Exhibits specific knowledge (grade 6).
- H: Can detect personal errors (grade 6).
- I: Describes and applies fitness principles (grade 6).

Standard 3: Participates Regularly in Physical Activity

Grades 3-5: Older children use conscious decision making to choose enjoyable activities that have health benefits. They can be active for longer periods and can identify opportunities for being active in a variety of settings. They use movement concepts to sustain enjoyable activity and regulate it.

Grade 6: Children participate in activities independently, set goals based on needs and interests, and apply practices and training principles. They participate in a broad range of activities and maintain an activity log.

Performance outcomes:

- A: Chooses activities that are enjoyable, and knows their benefits (grade 6).
- B: Participates for longer periods of time (grade 6).
- C: Chooses to participate in moderate to vigorous physical activity.
- D: Chooses to participate in structured and purposeful activity.
- E: Monitors physical activity.
- F: Maintains a physical activity log for two or three days.
- G: Participates independently (grade 6).
- H: Sets personal goals based on needs and interests (grade 6).
- I: Applies and practices activity principles (grade 6).
- J: Participates in a range of activities and maintains a log (grade 6).

Standard 4: Achieves and Maintains Health-Enhancing Physical Fitness

Grades 3-5: Older children participate in activity to improve fitness and can participate for a longer time without tiring. They do activity for health-related fitness and use physical indicators to monitor and make adjustments in activity. They take and learn about fitness tests as well as learn to interpret results with assistance.

Grade 6: Children participate in many activities without fatigue, know the components of and participate in activities for many parts of health-related fitness, and know the physical signs of exertion (e.g., heart rate, fast breathing, sweating). They can assess health-related fitness and interpret the results, set goals and monitor progress, and apply principles of training (overload, threshold, specificity).

Performance outcomes:

- A: Participates in selected activities to promote health-related fitness.
- B: Engages in activity that promotes cardiorespiratory fitness.
- C: Recognizes physical responses to activity associated with fitness.
- D: Participates in activities that build strength.
- E: Can explain consequences of poor flexibility.
- F: Maintains heart rate in target zone in aerobic activity.
- G: Meets age- and gender-specific health-related fitness standards.
- H: Identifies strengths and weaknesses on Fitnessgram tests.
- I: Participates in many activities.
- J: Knows parts of health-related fitness and participates in activities that promote them (grade 6).
- K: Can assess health-related fitness and interpret results (grades 5-6).
- L: Applies fitness principles (grade 6).
- M: Sets goals and monitors progress (grade 6).

Standard 5: Exhibits Responsible Personal and Social Behavior and Respect for Others in Activity

Grades 3-5: Older children are active and learn to work independently in groups and enjoy diversity in activity settings. They follow rules, safe practices, procedures, and etiquette. They continue to develop communication and cooperative skills. They continue to develop cultural and ethnic awareness and appreciate differences in others.

Grade 6: Children recognize the role of activity in understanding diversity, respect differences of others, and can move beyond just following rules to reflect on ethical behavior in cooperative and competitive activities. They work with greater independence, develop the ability to resolve conflicts, and use time wisely.

Performance outcomes:

- A: Cooperates with others in taking turns and sharing.
- B: Works productively with others in dance sequences.
- C: Accepts teacher's decisions without negative reactions.
- D: Takes responsibility for personal actions and does not blame others.
- E: Shows ability to communicate (grade 6).
- F: Works independently (grades 5-6).
- G: Recognizes and appreciates similarities and differences of activity choices in peers.
- H: Respects views of peers in discussion of differences in dances.
- I: Demonstrates respect for peers with disabilities.
- J: Encourages others and refrains from put-down statements.
- K: Uses ethical behavior in activity and cooperates in competition beyond following rules (grade 6).
- L: Works with greater independence and uses time wisely (grade 6).
- M: Helps resolve conflicts (grade 6).

Standard 6: Values Physical Activity for Health, Enjoyment, Challenge, Self-Expression, and Social Interaction

Grades 3-5: Older children can identify fun activities and are challenged by new skills and activities. They can associate good practice with learning of skills. They choose appropriate activities for their ability levels and engage in activity with students of differing abilities.

Grade 6: Children interact well in social situations, respect others and their abilities, and build self-confidence and self-esteem through improved performance resulting from practice.

Performance outcomes:

- A: Identifies positive feelings associated with participation in activity.
- B: Chooses to participate in group physical activities.
- C: Understands that skill competency aids enjoyment and regular participation.
- D: Interacts with others and helps others in activity.
- E: Selects and practices a skill that needs improvement.
- F: Develops a dance sequence that is enjoyable.
- G: Defends the benefits of activity.
- H: Identifies fun activities.
- I: Interacts well in social situations (grade 6).
- J: Respects others and their abilities (grade 6).
- K: Builds self-confidence through activity and improvement from practice (grade 6).

REFERENCES AND SUGGESTED RESOURCES

● ●

Beighle, A., Castelli, D., Erwin, H., & Ernst, M. (2009). Preparing physical educators for the role of physical activity director. *Journal of Physical Education Recreation and Dance, 80*(4), 24-28.

California Department of Education. (2003). *California physical fitness testing 2000: Report to the governor and legislature.* Sacramento, CA: California Department of Education.

California Department of Education. (2005). *California physical fitness testing 2002: Report to the governor and legislature.* Sacramento, CA: California Department of Education.

Castelli, D., Hillman, C.H., Buck, S.M., & Erwin, H.E. (2006). Physical fitness and academic Achievement in third- and fifth-grade students. *Journal of Exercise and Sport Psychology, 28*(3), 239-252.

Chomitz, V.R., Slining, M.M., McGowan, R.J., Mitchell, S.E., Dawson, G.F., & Hacker, K.A. (2009). Is there a relationship between physical fitness and academic achievement? Positive results from public school children in the Northeastern United States. *Journal of School Health, 79,* 30-37.

Dwyer, T., Sallis, J.F., Blizzard, L., Lazarus, R., & Dean, K. (2001). Relationship of academic performance to physical activity and fitness in children. *Pediatric Exercise Science, 13,* 225-237.

Ernst, M.P., Corbin, C.B., Beighle, A., & Pangrazi, R.P. (2006). Appropriate and inappropriate uses of FITNESSGRAM: A commentary. *Journal of Physical Activity and Health, 3*(Supplement), S90-S100.

Field, T., Diego, M., & Sanders, C.E. (2001). Exercise is positively related to adolescents' relationships and academics. *Adolescence, 36*(141), 105-110.

Gabbard, C., & Barton, J. (1979). Effects of physical activity on mathematical computation among young children. *Journal of Psychology, 103,* 287-288.

Grissom, J.B. (2005). Physical fitness and academic achievement. *Journal of Exercise Physiology, 8*(1), 11-25.

Hillman, C.H., Buck, S.M., Themanson, J.R., Pontifex, M.B., & Castelli, D. (2009a). Aerobic fitness and cognitive development: Event-related brain potential and task performance indices of executive control in preadolescent children. *Developmental Psychology, 45,* 114-129.

Hillman, C.H., Pontifex, M.B., Raine, L.B., Castelli, D.M., Hall, E.E., & Kramer, A.F. (2009b). The effect of acute treadmill walking on cognitive control and academic achievement in preadolescent children. *Neuroscience, 159,* 1044-1054.

Le Masurier, G.C., & Corbin, C.B. (2006). Top 10 reasons for quality physical education. *Journal of Physical Education Recreation and Dance, 77*(6), 44-53.*nce, 159,* 1044-1054.

McNaughton, D., & Gabbard, C. (1993). Physical exertion and immediate mental performance of sixth grade children. *Perceptual Motor Skills, 77* (3 pt. 2), 1155-1159.

NASPE. (1998). *Physical activity for children: A statement of guidelines.* Reston, VA: Author.

NASPE. (2004a). *Moving into the future: National standards for physical education.* Reston, VA: Author.

NASPE. (2004b). *Physical activity for children: A statement of guidelines for children 5-12.* Reston, VA: Author.

NASPE. (2004c). *Physical Best activity guide: Elementary level.* 2nd ed. Champaign, IL: Human Kinetics.

Ogden, C.L., Carroll, M.D., & Flegal, K.M. (2008). High body mass index for age among U.S. children and adolescents, 2003-2006. *Journal of the American Medical Association, 299*(20), 2401-2405.*nce, 159,* 1044-1054.

Pangrazi, R.P. (2006). *Active and healthy schools program.* Owatonna, MN: Gopher.

Pate, R.R., Baranowski, T., Dowda, M., & Trost, S.G. (1996). Tracking of physical activity in young children. *Medicine and Science in Sports and Exercise, 28*(1), 92-96.

Ratey, J.J. (2008). *SPARK: The revolutionary new science of exercise and the brain.* New York: Little, Brown and Co.

Sallis, J.F., McKenzie, T.L., Kolody, B., Lewis, M., Marshall, S., & Rosengard, P. (1999). Effects of health-related physical education on academic achievement: Project SPARK. *Research Quarterly for Exercise and Sport, 70*(2), 127-134.

Serdula, M.K., Ivery, D., Coates, R.J., Freedman, D.S., Williamson, D.F., & Byers, T. (1993). Do obese children become obese adults? A review of the literature. *Preventative Medicine, 22,* 167-177.

Shephard, R.J., Lavallee, H., Volle, M., LaBarre, R., & Beaucage, C. (1994). Academic skills and required physical education: The Trois Rivieres experience. *Canadian Association for Health, Physical Education, and Recreation, Suppl. 1*(1), 1-12.

Shephard, R.J., Lavallee, H., Volle, M., LaBarre, R., & Beaucage, C. (1997). Curricular physical activity and academic performance. *Pediatric Exercise Science, 9,* 113-126.

Shephard, R.J., & Trudeau, F. (2005). Lessons learned from the Trois-Rivieres physical education study: A retrospective. *Pediatric Exercise Science, 17*(2), 112-113.

Sibley, B.A., & Etnier, J.L. (2003). The relationship between physical activity and cognition in children: A meta-analysis. *Pediatric Exercise Science, 15,* 243-256.

Sibley, B.A., Etnier, J.L., Pangrazi, R.P., & Le Masurier, G.C. (2006). Effects of acute bouts of physical activity on inhibition and cognitive performance. *Journal of Sport and Exercise Psychology, 28*(3), 285-299.

Smith, N.J., & Lounsbery, M. (2009). Promoting physical education: The link to academic achievement. *Journal of Physical Education, Recreation and Dance, 80*(1), 39-43.

Strong, W., Malina, R., Blimkie, C., Daniels, S., Dishman, B., Gutin, B., Hergenroeder, A., Must, A., Nixon, P., & Pivarnik, J. (2005). Evidence-based physical activity for school-age youth. *Journal of Pediatrics, 146*(6), 732-737.

Trudeau, F., Laurencelle, L., Tremblay, J., Rajic, M., & Shephard, R.J. (1998). A long-term follow-up of participants in the Trois-Rivieres semi-longitudinal study of growth and development. *Pediatric Exercise Science, 10*(4), 366-377.

Trudeau, F., & Shephard, R.J. (2005). Contribution of school programmes to physical activity levels and attitudes in children and adults. *Sports Medicine, 35*(2), 89-105.

USDA. (2005). Daily guidelines for Americans—2005. Washington, DC: Author (access at www.health.gov/DietaryGuidelines/).

USDHHS. (2008). 2008 Physical activity guidelines for Americans: Be active, healthy, and happy. Washington, DC: Author (access at www.health.gov/paguidelines/guidelines/default.aspx).

Whitaker, R.C., Wright, J.A., Pepe, M.S., Seidel, K.D., & Dietz, W.H. (1997). Predicting obesity in young adulthood from childhood and parental obesity. *New England Journal of Medicine, 37*(13), 869-873.*nce, 159,* 1044-1054.

World Health Organization (WHO). (1947). Constitution of the World Health Organization. *Chronicle of the World Health Organization, 1,* 29-43.

Web Resources

Note: The Web addresses below are from credible organizations. From time to time, organizations change names or Web site addresses. If a link below does not work, searching the Web for the name of the organization will often lead you to the information you are looking for.

Fitness for Life: Elementary School: www.fitnessforlife.org (click on Elementary)

MyPyramid: www.MyPyramid.gov

Action for Healthy Kids: www.actionforhealthykids.org

American Association for Physical Activity and Recreation: www.aahperd.org/aapar/

Body Mass Index (BMI) Calculator: http://apps.nccd.cdc.gov/dnpabmi

Centers for Disease Prevention and Control (CDC) Additional youth overweight and obesity: www.cdc.gov/nccdphp/dnpa/obesity/childhood/defining.htm

Educational Standards for All subjects: www.educationworld.com/standards/national/toc/index.shtml#lang

National Health Observances: www.healthfinder.gov

National Language Arts Standards (National Council of Teachers of English NCTE): www1.ncte.org/store/books/bestsellers/105977.htm?source=gs

National Math Standards (National Council of Teachers of Mathematics): www.nctm.org/standards/focalpoints.aspx?id=298

National Nutrition Month: www.jimcolemanltd.com/nnm/

National P.E. and Sports Week (National Association for Sports and Physical Education): www.aahperd.org/Naspe/MayWeek/2009/template.cfm?template=main.htm

National Science Standards: http://www.nsta.org/publications/nses.aspx and www.educationworld.com/standards/national/toc/index.shtml#science

National Social Studies Standards: www.socialstudies.org/standards/taskforce/fall2008draft

President's Council on Physical Fitness and Sports: www.fitness.gov

Project ACES (All Children Exercising Simultaneously): http://lensaunders.com/aces/aces.html

School Breakfast (School Nutrition Association): www.schoolnutrition.org

Texas Physical Fitness Study: www.ourkidshealth.org

Turn Off (the TV) Week: http://247moms.blogspot.com/2009/04/national-turn-off-tv-week-unplug-your.html

USDA: Child Nutrition Act of 2004: www.fns.usda.gov/TN/Healthy/108-265.pdf

USDA General Web site: www.usda.gov/wps/portal/usdahome

USDA Nutrition Guidelines: www.health.gov/DietaryGuidelines/

Walk to School: www.walktoschool-usa.org

ABOUT THE AUTHORS

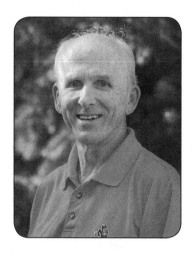

Charles B. "Chuck" Corbin, PhD, is currently professor emeritus in the department of exercise and wellness at Arizona State University. He has published more than 200 journal articles and is the senior author of, sole author of, contributor to, or editor of more than 80 books, including the 5th edition of *Fitness for Life* (winner of the TAA's Texty Award), the 14th edition of *Concepts of Physical Fitness* (winner of the TAA's McGuffey Award), and the 7th edition of *Concepts of Fitness and Wellness*. His books are the most widely adopted high school and college texts in fitness and wellness. Dr. Corbin is internationally recognized as an expert in physical activity, health and wellness promotion, and youth physical fitness. He has presented keynote addresses at more than 40 state AHPERD conventions, made major addresses in more than 15 countries, and presented numerous named lectures (Cureton, ACSM; Hanna, Sargent, and Distinguished Scholar, NAKPEHE; Prince Phillip, British PEA; and Weiss and Alliance Scholar, AAHPERD). He is past president and fellow of AAKPE, fellow in the NASHPERDP, an ACSM fellow, and a lifetime member of AAHPERD. Among his awards are the Healthy American Fitness Leaders Award (President's Council on Physical Fitness and Sports—PCPFS, National Jaycees), AAHPERD Honor Award, Physical Fitness Council Honor Award, the COPEC Hanson Award, and the Distinguished Service Award of the PCPFS. Dr. Corbin was named the Alliance Scholar by AAHPERD and the Distinguished Scholar of NAKPEHE. He is a member of the Fitnessgram Advisory Board and was the first chair of the science board of the PCPFS and the NASPE Hall of Fame. In 2009 Dr. Corbin was chosen for the Gulick Award, the highest award of AAHPERD.

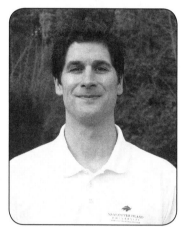

Guy Le Masurier, PhD, is a professor of physical education at Vancouver Island University, where he teaches courses in pedagogy, research methods, and nutrition for health and sport. Dr. Le Masurier is coauthor of the award-winning book *Fitness for Life: Middle School* (winner of the TAA's Texty Award) and has edited and contributed to several books, including the 5th edition of *Fitness for Life* and the *Physical Best Activity Guide*. He has published numerous articles related to youth physical activity and physical education and served as a coauthor on the *NASPE Physical Activity Guidelines for Children*. Dr. Le Masurier has delivered over 30 research and professional presentations at national and regional meetings and currently serves as the Epidemiology section editor for *Research Quarterly for Exercise and Sport* as well as the Health Foundations section editor for the *International Journal of Physical Education*. Dr. Le Masurier is the creator of the Walk Everyday Live Longer (WELL) program, a pedometer-based physical activity program used by the Arizona Department of Health Services. Dr. Le Masurier is a member of AAHPERD, NASPE, and ACSM. He lives with his wife on Protection Island in British Columbia, where they serve their community as volunteer firefighters. Guy is thankful for his morning kayak commutes.

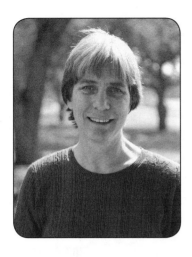

Dolly D. Lambdin, EdD, is a senior lecturer in the department of kinesiology and health education at the University of Texas at Austin, where she teaches undergraduate courses in children's movement and methods of teaching as well as graduate courses in analysis of teaching and technology application in physical education.

Dr. Lambdin taught elementary physical education in public and private schools for 16 years and taught preservice teachers for 33 years at the university level. During much of that time, she taught simultaneously at both levels, a situation that required her to spend part of each day meeting the teaching and research demands of academia while tackling the daily adventure of teaching 5- to 14-year-olds. In addition, she has supervised over 100 student teachers, and as a result has been able to visit classes and learn from scores of wonderful cooperating teachers in the schools.

Dr. Lambdin has served as the president of NASPE (2004-05) and on the NASPE board of directors for two three-year terms. She has also served on numerous local, state, and national committees, including the writing teams for the Texas Essential Knowledge and Skills in Physical Education, the NASPE Beginning Teacher Standards, the Texas Beginning Teacher Standards, and the NASPE Appropriate Practices Revision. Dr. Lambdin has been honored as the Texas AHPERD Outstanding College and University Physical Educator of the Year.

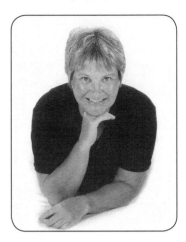

Meg Greiner, MEd, is a national board-certified elementary physical education teacher at Independence Elementary School in Independence, Oregon. She has been teaching elementary physical education for 21 years and regularly receives student teachers and practicum students into her setting. Meg has received numerous national awards and accolades for her innovative physical education program and the development of TEAM Time, including the 2005 NASPE National Elementary Physical Education Teacher of the Year, 2005 *USA Today* All-USA Teacher Team, and the 2006 Disney Outstanding Specialist Teacher of the Year. Meg is currently working with NASPE as a Head Start Body Start trainer of trainers, serving on the AAHPERD Physical Best Committee, and presenting NASPE Pipeline Workshops all over the United States. She has served on the NASPE Council of Physical Education for Children and on the public relations committee. She has served as the physical education president for both Oregon and Northwest District AHPERDs. She also has served Oregon AHPERD in many capacities and has received the OAHPERD Honor Award.

DVD USER INSTRUCTIONS

The DVD-ROM contains videos and resources for the wellness coordinator to use when implementing the **Fitness for Life: Elementary School** program.

Videos

When you insert the disc in a DVD player, the TV screen displays the following Main Menu:

- TEAM Time 1
- TEAM Time 2
- TEAM Time 3
- TEAM Time 4
- Interview with Chuck Corbin
- Resources
- Credits

Part II of this book walks you through the steps for planning each Wellness Week and instructs you when to play the appropriate videos for each TEAM Time activity. You can play the interview with Chuck Corbin, senior author of **Fitness for Life**, when presenting the program to school staff.

Resources

The resources can be viewed only on a computer with a DVD-ROM drive. To access the resources, follow the instructions below for Microsoft Windows® or Macintosh® computers.

Microsoft Windows

1. Place the DVD in the DVD-ROM drive of your computer.
2. Double-click on the "My Computer" icon from your desktop.
3. Right-click on the DVD-ROM drive and select the "Open" option from the pop-up menu.
4. Open the Resources folder and then the General folder or one of the Wellness Week folders to find the desired resource.
5. Select the file you want to view and print.

Macintosh

1. Place the DVD in the DVD-ROM drive of your computer.
2. Double-click on the DVD icon on your desktop.
3. Open the Resources folder and then the General folder or one of the Wellness Week folders to find the desired resource.
4. Select the file that you want to view and print.

You will need Adobe® Reader® to view the PDF files.